Emotional

INFERTILITY

LEAH LLOYD

National Library of Australia Cataloguing-in-Publication data:
Leah Lloyd/Emotional Infertility
Non-Fiction– Infertility

Editor: Natasha Gilmour
Proofreader: Teena Raffa-Mulligan
Cover and interior designer: Ida Jansson

Dedicated to Isabelle and Charlotte.
May the choice always be yours,
thank you for being my greatest achievement.
Love, Mum. xx

Contents

Introduction   7
How It All Began   10
How To Use This Book   15
Tapping The Healer Within   18
Meditation for Fertility   21
Before We Begin   23
   Journaling: meeting your emotional self   24
   Meditation: for body gratitude   25

CHAPTER ONE: UNDERSTANDING YOUR CYCLE   31
   Journaling: reflection activity   38
   Meditation: for physical reproductive ailments   39

CHAPTER TWO: UNDERSTANDING INFERTILITY CAUSES   43
   Journaling: fertility considerations   52
   Tapping Script 1: for fear you did something wrong   53
   Meditation: for improving health   56

CHAPTER THREE: TUNING IN TO YOUR EMOTIONS   60
   Journaling: embrace your emotional self   64
   Meditation: for motherhood   66

CHAPTER FOUR: HOW FEELINGS EFFECT FERTILITY   69
   Journaling: clearing emotions by clearing the mind   73
   Tapping Script 2: for jealousy of other people having babies   76
   Meditation: for feeling joy when you see a baby   80

CHAPTER FIVE: BELIEFS ON YOUR ABILITY TO BE A PARENT   84
   Journaling: drawing out your feelings   87
   Meditation: for ability to parent   88

CHAPTER SIX: EMOTIONS AS ENERGY   91
   Journaling: changing your vibration   94
   Meditation: for support   95

CHAPTER SEVEN: EMOTIONAL AWARENESS   99
   Journaling: feelings for pregnancy   101

CHAPTER EIGHT: FINDING HAPPINESS BEFORE THE BABY   102
   Journaling: identifying feelings for happiness   106

CHAPTER NINE: RELEASING STRESS AND GUILT   108
   Journal: writing out stressors and guilt   116

Tapping Script 3: for stress   117

CHAPTER TEN: RELATIONSHIPS FOR FERTILITY   119
Journaling: for fertile grounds   121

CHAPTER ELEVEN: SINGLE WOMEN AND SAME-SEX COUPLES   123
Journaling: for clarity on your fertility path   126

CHAPTER TWELVE: IVF, DONORS AND SURROGACY   127
Journaling: for acceptance; thoughts, beliefs   131
Meditation: for IVF   132
Meditation: for IVF embryo transfer   136
Meditation: for embryos being transferred into a surrogate   139
Meditation: for a surrogate   142

CHAPTER THIRTEEN: ABUSE AND TRAUMA   146
Journaling: for abuse therapy   149

CHAPTER FOURTEEN: CULTURAL CONSIDERATIONS   150
Journaling: for cultural awareness   153

CHAPTER FIFTEEN: SECONDARY INFERTILITY   154
Journaling: shifting perspectives for baby 2   156

CHAPTER SIXTEEN: FERTILITY AFTER MISCARRIAGE, ABORTION
OR A STILLBORN   157
Journaling: to heal the womb   160
Tapping Script 4: for trying for a baby after having lost one   162
Meditation: for previous miscarriages   165
Meditation: for previous abortions   168
Meditation: for a previous stillborn   171

CHAPTER SEVENTEEN: WHAT ABOUT THE MEN   174
Journaling: for him   176

CHAPTER EIGHTEEN: WHAT IF I'M NO LONGER INFERTILE?   177
Journaling: writing for a positive pregnancy   180
Tapping Script 5: for once you are pregnant   182

CHAPTER NINETEEN: ACCEPTING I WILL NEVER BE A MOTHER   186
Tapping Script 5: for acceptance   188

Emotional resources toolkit   **191**
Affirmations   **191**
Essential Oils   **193**
Further Resources   **195**
Bibliography   **197**

Introduction

Before you begin, I want you to know this: <u>It Is Not Your Fault</u>.

You didn't do anything wrong, and you don't 'deserve' infertility. If you are blaming yourself for anything, start to address it as you work through this book. You can't be responsible for what you didn't know. As you work through this book and learn and understand, you will become empowered. Helping you to make decisions that are right for you and letting go of what no longer serves you, beliefs, blame, guilt or anger.

It is my intention through this book that every woman becomes educated—you can heal any aspect of oneself needed—giving you the best chance of achieving a pregnancy, either naturally or using assisted reproductive technology.

For this book, we will be mostly looking at women's infertility, but the concepts also apply to men, and I would encourage any man experiencing infertility to address the issues outlined in this book.

If you are in a relationship and having fertility issues, it may be helpful to go through this process together. Sadly, relationships can break down during such a difficult time, and it is important to take steps to stay united in the process together.

This book does not replace seeing your medical doctor and seeking treatment and assistance in achieving and maintaining a pregnancy. Always follow the guidance of your doctor or specialist.

The goal of this book is simply for you to look at some possible reasons you may be experiencing infertility and identify any *emotional* causes behind them. We very rarely realise the effects our personal or learned beliefs have on our physical bodies, as well as the effects of the experiences that have led you to this moment. By addressing these issues, you give yourself the best chance of achieving a spontaneous pregnancy, or through assisted reproductive techniques, such as insemination or IVF. By looking at an illness or disease, and seeing how it works, gives us clues as to why these physical issues appear in the body. In my experience, two of the most common female fertility issues are Polycystic Ovaries (PCOS) and endometriosis. PCOS is an endocrine disturbance characterised by a lack of ovulation, irregular or no periods, increased hair growth and infertility. Medically, PCOS is caused by increased levels of oestrogen, testosterone and luteinising hormone (LH), and decreased secretion of follicle stimulating hormone (FSH). The depressed but continuous production of FSH causes continuous development of ovarian follicles, resulting in the affected ovary doubling in size and containing many cysts (Anderson, 1998, p1289). PCOS affects approximately a quarter of women of child-bearing age (IVFA).

Inna Segal is an award-winning best-selling author of *The Secret Language of Your Body: The Essential Guide to Health and Wellness*, she suggests ovarian cysts mean, 'holding onto old hurts from men and pain from previous abuse, mental, emotional or physical. 'Segal states, 'Ovarian cysts can indicate not feeling good enough, rejecting your femininity, fertility problems, hiding sadness and disappointment, feeling unloved and lonely, or conflict with female relatives or friends.'

Endometriosis is defined as an abnormal gynaecologic condition characterised by abnormal growth and function of endometrial tissue. It is suspected the condition is largely undiagnosed, partially due to the difficulty in diagnosing it;

however, approximately 15% of women in the US who undergo pelvic laparotomy for other indications are found to have endometriosis. In Australia, around 10% of women are known to have endometriosis, and it is most common in women over thirty that haven't yet had children (IVFA). Segal states, 'that endometriosis results from feeling inadequate, unacceptable and not good enough. Rejecting the feminine aspect of yourself, feeling depleted, unsupported or ungrounded. Holding on to feelings of rejection from others, especially men. Devaluing and dishonouring yourself. Denying yourself love and appreciation.'

There is no guarantee that by working through this process you will become pregnant. I wish I could give you that, but there are so many factors to fertility. This book will focus mostly on the *emotional* aspects. Seeing a fertility specialist and taking the appropriate steps with them may also be a vital part of this journey for you.

I hope this book brings you healing, guidance and acceptance. I wish you every success on this journey.

How It All Began

"I am not defined by my story."

Growing up, I knew I wanted to be a mum more than anything else.

I started babysitting as soon as I was old enough and mothered my little sister. I put her back in her cot when she climbed out, taught her to swim and showed her how to drive a car.

When I became a nurse, I managed to convince my preceptor in my post-graduate year to let me do a rotation in maternity. They called me back for shifts often, which I loved. I particularly liked caring for the babies in the special care nursery. There was one baby boy whose mum was unable to visit much, and I would pick him up and feed him, and cuddle him that extra little bit longer, so he knew he was loved.

During my post-graduate year, I was admitted to hospital to have my appendix removed. However, after the procedure was done the surgeon said there was nothing wrong with my appendix. There must have been another cause for the pain I had been experiencing.

A few months later, I had an ultrasound and blood tests, and was told I had Polycystic Ovarian Syndrome (PCOS). With over twenty cysts on my right ovary it explained the pain I had been having, my irregular periods and several other symptoms. I remember clearly my GP telling me, 'Have your babies before you turn 26 or you won't have them.' I was 21 at the time, and in my first

10

year of nursing. It was *not* a good time to consider having children. I remember feeling torn—I wanted this more than anything—but now I had a time limit and my circumstances would not allow for me to stop work and have a baby. I was devastated to say the least.

Fortunately, I was in a happy marriage, and after a lot of discussion we started 'trying'. I actually thought I would get pregnant easily because I was young and healthy. In my mind, I saw the situation as an excuse to be allowed to have a baby now. I didn't think it would be hard.

However, month-after-month when my period came, I lost a little more of my spirit. None of my friends were looking at having children then and didn't understand what I was going through. My sister had her first baby at this time, and I babysat him every chance I got. If I wasn't at work I was looking after my nephew, and I loved every minute.

My husband, however, became more distant, enjoying the life of a young person, while all I wanted was to work on improving my diet and increasing my chances of becoming pregnant. I changed my diet considerably to low GI, and this helped regulate my periods somewhat. Excitedly, I told my husband that I was pretty sure if we had sex every day for a particular week, it should cover the day I ovulate and we should get pregnant. My husband made an excuse every day that week to *not* have sex with me. And that was the beginning of the end of my marriage. We both had different priorities then. I moved out and we divorced the following year. So now I had a time limit and no husband. I became depressed.

I blamed my body mostly, how could it betray me like this? I blamed myself for all of those years of being on the pill, or for praying not to get pregnant in a previous bad relationship. I put on weight, I drank too much, I was really not interested in myself or my future at that point. I lacked support as none of my friends understood why I'd left my marriage (when people are just getting married, they don't want any reminders that it might not work out). I enjoyed my work and that got me through, but I didn't want to work in maternity anymore. I couldn't face seeing those little babies, knowing that was not in my future. I begrudged the young girls down the street with their prams and cigarettes hanging out their mouths, they didn't even appreciate what they had, or how lucky they were to have it. They didn't deserve it, but I did, and I couldn't have it. It was a very bitter pill to swallow. I was struggling.

Amazingly, after meeting my new husband, I became pregnant without any effort whatsoever. I had given up being careful, resigned to the fact that I was *infertile*. I have always had a strong belief in things happening as they are meant to, and I firmly believe this was one of those times. My beautiful daughter is proof of that. My second daughter came along just as easily and unplanned, the day after my first daughters second birthday. I always thought I would have baby number three, twins were my plan: a boy and a girl. I was sure when we started 'trying' again it would happen as easily as my other pregnancies, but it wasn't to be. My period completely stopped for six months, and I had to go back on the pill to regulate them, this was the only solution my GP could offer. I wanted a baby though, and this was not going to make it happen. So, I went off the pill and changed my diet again, this time paleo, and got my periods to roughly a 35-45-day cycle. Anyone who has tried for a baby knows the little glimmer of hope that lives in your heart every time your period is late. One component of PCOS is that it can make your period late How cruel that was. I had forgotten how painful the monthly reminder of getting your period was, and the sinking feeling that went with it. I couldn't go through that again.

During this time, I trained in Energy Healing. I was seeing clients with physical reasons for not getting pregnant or keeping a pregnancy, but there was often an emotional cause behind the physical cause. Given my own history, I found this incredibly interesting, and my original interest in babies was sparked once again. I became excited about working in the field, instead of it being a painful reminder of what I hadn't achieved.

Our final year of trying was the year I turned 35. Mostly, I was working in an unhappy environment, my health was suffering, and I knew I needed to make some changes. But to change jobs for a better lifestyle meant a reduction in pay and a commitment to that new job. Nevertheless, my husband and I made the decision that we were done trying and happy with our family of four and I took my new job at a fertility clinic.

This job led to me becoming a teacher in natural fertility. I was shocked to learn so much about my body I had never known. Why wasn't I taught this when I was first diagnosed with PCOS? Why wasn't I taught this when I was put on the pill? Or when I had my first period? Long before that would have been even better. It is every woman's right to know her body, to understand it and what it is telling her. Every woman should be empowered with this information, not taught to fear it, or be controlled by a lack of knowledge. Make it your priority to be empowered through research and understanding. Know the basics and track your cycles. Then work your way through this book, reading every chapter and doing the activities. Through knowledge and self-growth, you will be empowered.

I was lucky that I had both of my children naturally in the end. But I will never forget that feeling of not being able to have kids. The feeling that the choice had been pulled out from under me, I had lost my footing. As a woman it was my right to have a child if I wanted one, surely. My choice to make. Every month my period came, I felt like someone had punched me in the guts. Like it was a cruel joke I was the subject of. It was an overwhelming and heartbreaking experience that I wouldn't wish upon anyone. That is why 'I get it' and why I want to help.

Interestingly, after making the decision to not have our third child, I discovered dōTERRA essential oils, specifically the women's monthly blend. For the first time in my life I have a regular cycle and my symptoms have settled down. I honestly believe if I tried again now, I would have a chance of success. However, the journey of writing this book has also been healing for me in addressing my beliefs and emotions, and I actually feel okay about not having another child at this stage of my life.

I believe the other big factor not only for creating better health in general, but also fertile cycles, is managing stress. I was always a stressed-out person. The workload at school and university with fitting in part time jobs always felt tiring. Then going on to nursing, and then trying to fit in a family, managing my health and trying to have a life in addition to all of this felt overwhelming. I'm sure this was a big contributor to my failing health at the time and for my periods stopping altogether. Discovering meditation, yoga and Tai Chi has been a life saver for me. I have dedicated a whole chapter to stress in this book because I am so sure it is one of the biggest contributing factors to infertility *and* every other health problem out there.

Not everyone will read my book and go on to have a child, but I believe in my heart that many will. I hope this book can also bring you some comfort and healing.

How To Use This Book

"Today, I take back my power."

My aim in writing this book is to give you the opportunity to *emotionally* heal yourself. I'm sharing with you the processes, clearing techniques, tapping scripts, meditations and insights that have helped my clients on their personal fertility journey. If you find you need more specific help with your emotions, please see a professional therapist. Emotions can become big and overwhelming particularly when going through something as significant and difficult as infertility, so it can be very helpful to have someone to talk through the process with.

I have created a beautiful *Emotional Infertility Companion Workbook* to use while you read this book. There are journaling activities at the end of each chapter to help you positively heal. Perhaps some may be difficult at certain times on your journey, so please seek help if needed throughout the process. Generally, the activities that seem to be the most difficult to face, will be the ones that bring you the most healing. Writing and getting all of your feelings out on paper can be beneficial and rewarding. By writing the words there is an acknowledgement of your feelings. It is also a safe place to express anger or resentment that you may not want to inflict on someone you love, but still need to get it out. I recommend keeping it somewhere safe. If you know it won't be read by anyone else you will feel free to write as honestly as possible, and this is where true healing can happen. Each journaling activity will also give you information to use for tapping or creating affirmations.

I guide you to read the book first, then come back to the beginning and take your time working through the pages with your *Companion Workbook*. You may also need to re-visit some chapters as your journey unfolds.

Throughout this book, I will ask you to use tools such as *affirmations* and *Emotional Freedom Technique*, also known as EFT or tapping. When using affirmations or the positive statements in EFT, sometimes it won't feel 'true' and that can alter the effectiveness. I have found the easiest way to overcome this is to acknowledge it right at the beginning. In your journal you might like to write something like:

> 'Even though I know there is no guarantee I will have a baby at the end of this journey, and I know there is a chance that these affirmations won't be the reality in the end. I am going to do them anyway and I'm going to give it all I've got. I can deal with any other possible outcomes if and when the need arises.'

This way you are acknowledging that the affirmations are not yet your reality in some instances; however, when you are saying them you are not 'lying' or 'pretending' but giving yourself the greatest chance of making them true. If you still struggle with the idea, you can always add: 'I choose ...' or 'I will ...' at the beginning of the affirmation or positive statements.

This book is in no way diagnostic; however, I feel that the emotional aspects and impacts of infertility are often overlooked. If you have any of the physical symptoms mentioned throughout the book, please have a check-up with your general practitioner to ensure everything is in order. This is a good idea before getting pregnant anyway. Your doctor will review any medications you're on, make sure your vaccinations are up-to-date if you have them, discuss any health concerns you might have and possibly run some baseline blood tests.

Tapping The Healer Within

"I have the ability to heal myself."

EFT (Emotional Freedom Technique) fondly known as *tapping* is an incredibly easy technique to use. It is effective, free and you can do it anywhere. I have created a tapping script at the end of some chapters for you, depending on your circumstances some may be more useful than others. You can change the wording to suit your needs, or if you feel comfortable following the format I have created, make up your own script.

Before you start your first tapping session, spend a moment just sitting with your emotions—identify your stress levels of 0 to 10—zero being *no* stress and 10 being overwhelming stress. If you struggle to come up with a number ask yourself, 'do I feel less or more than an average stress,' then go above or below five. The actual number isn't so important, it's that the level of stress is decreasing as you tap that is important.

You will start with tapping 'The Karate Chop' point on the base of your hand down from your little finger. You will repeat the set-up statement or variations of the statement three times.

From here you will move through the 8 points shown in the picture below saying your negative statements as you tap on each point. Do as many cycles of this as you need to until your stress is less than two, or the negative statements are no longer feeling true for you.

When you feel ready to move on, continue to tap through

points 1-8 but start saying your positive statements. If they don't feel like you are being honest, you can add, 'I choose to…' or 'I wonder if…' or 'Maybe…' at the beginning. Keep going with the positives until you can lose these starting comments, or until they feel true for you.

Check in with how you're feeling when you think about the situation you just worked on. Is there any stress now when you think about it and if so, is it improved from before you started? Sometimes when you tap you start to think of other things that need to be addressed, other aspects of a situation, or feelings you hadn't identified or acknowledged previously. This will likely be an ongoing process that you will need to revisit, but it's free, it's easy and it's really worth it, so stick with it.

Sometimes when we haven't been given a good education around something as important as our menstrual cycle, we can feel angry or hurt, creating emotional infertility blocks on our journey. Throughout this book, explore any issues that come up for you and use the tapping activity provided to process and create new beliefs, such as:

'I am empowered and have some control over what is happening.'

As you do the exercises throughout the book you will have a lot of information ready to use for your tapping. I find it useful to go through your journal and in one colour highlight the perceived 'negatives' and in another colour the 'positives'.

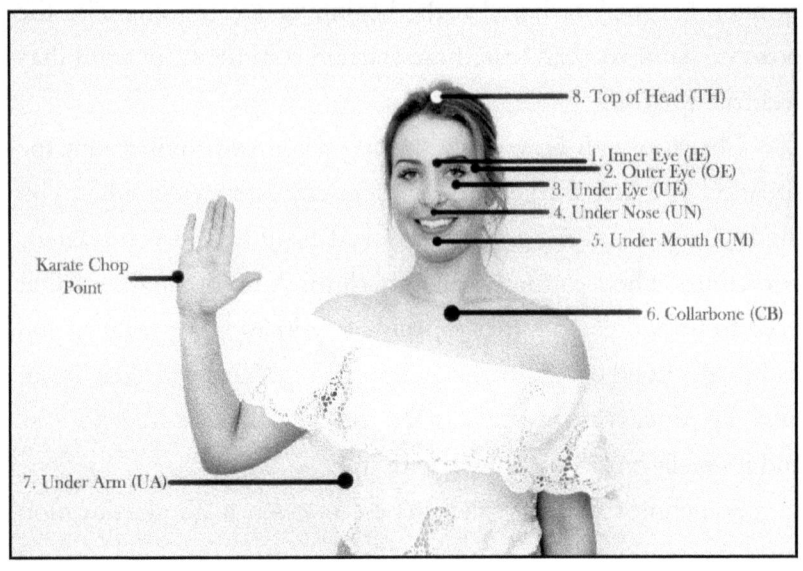

Where to tap

1. Inner Eyebrow (IE)
2. Outer Eye (OE)
3. Under Eye (UE)
4. Under Nose (UN)
5. Under Mouth (UM)
6. Collarbone (CB) *Use fist*
7. Under Arm (UA) *Use hand*
8. Top of the Head (TH)
9. The karate chop point (KP) *Use four fingers*

Meditation for Fertility

"I connect with the healer within me."

Meditation can be a very foreign concept to some people. I know when I first studied meditation and I had to do it without the help of a guided audio. I thought it would be impossible. But with time and practice it became easier. The more you do it, the more you will see the benefits. If it becomes a habit, you will use it even on your hardest days, when you need it most, but it seems the most difficult time to sit still.

I have written several guided meditations here for varying issues. You might find some more helpful than others. Perhaps it will be most helpful to record the words and then listen to the audio as you meditate. You might also like to try writing and recording your own meditations so it's specific to your circumstances. If sitting still and listening is difficult some days, there are other forms of meditation such as moving meditations you might find easier.

Before you relax into any of these meditations, be sure you are in a quiet place, where you won't be interrupted. You might like to dim the lights or burn a candle. If you would like to diffuse essential oils or have the fragrance of fresh flowers, prepare these before continuing. Relaxation music can also be very beneficial when meditating and is readily available on YouTube.

Most of the meditations use a different relaxation method, so you can pick and choose which ones resonate for you. It would be worth trying all of them though, so you can see which ones work best for you. Relaxation is vital for meditation to be effective, so don't rush through this part even if it's tempting.

If you are new to meditation you might fall asleep and this is okay. Simply repeat the meditation again at another time. Drink plenty of water when meditating and keep your journal nearby so you can write down any insights that come to you.

When you are ready to start, gently lie down on the floor, on a mat or rug. You might like to place a pillow under your head, and under your knees if it is comfortable. You might like a blanket to keep you warm. Allow your body to relax into a comfortable position, resting gently against the floor, allowing your feet to drop outwards. Your arms are relaxing gently beside your body, palms facing upwards. If you would prefer you can sit in a chair that supports your back, or cross-legged on the floor.

Before We Begin

"I commit to showing my body unconditional love and gratitude every day."

Before you begin, I encourage you to start your *Emotional Infertility* journey by watching the tapping script I have recorded for you, followed by a guided mediation *for body gratitude*—a powerful combination—to set your highest intentions towards your *emotional* healing.

It is important to *meet your emotional self* in the journaling activity below before you read through the pages on how your cycle works in chapter one, even if you think you have a thorough understanding of it. You don't know what you don't know and there could be something vital that you haven't learnt before. Knowing how your body works is a really important basis for everything else. It eliminates a lot of the second guessing and the fear around infertility.

When I studied women's health at university, the lecturer who worked as a women's health nurse saw a lot of clients with infertility. Many of them were doing basic things that stopped them getting pregnant such as taking the pill (they were on the pill to regulate their cycles, to prevent having a period or to manage their acne and hadn't thought about the fact it was also stopping them from getting pregnant). Not to be crass here, but to make the point that not everyone is well educated on their anatomy. Another person was having anal intercourse with the assumption everything met up inside where it should. So, don't assume because you did sex education at school that you have a good understanding and even if you do it won't hurt to have a quick refresher.

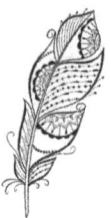

Journaling: meeting your emotional self

Start by writing 'your story' as I have above in the introduction *How It All Began*. This writing is just for you, so be as honest as possible. Use whatever language feels right. Don't worry about spelling, punctuation or grammar. The important thing here is to be true to you with what you write, to allow yourself to feel and heal.

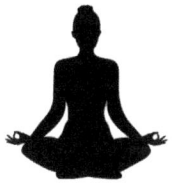

Meditation: for body gratitude

Often when we are going through infertility, we start to blame our body for not working. This is a normal response, but it can be damaging if it lasts for a long period of time. We don't tend to look after something we don't appreciate. Our body is an amazing arrangement of intricate systems, that all need to work together to function effectively. Often it needs to do this with poor nutrient intake, high levels of stress, and unfavourable environmental influences. By using this meditation regularly, you will become more and more grateful for the body you have, and in turn will treat it better, which can only influence your *fertility* positively.

This meditation focuses on the whole body and is suitable for both men and women. And, is best done lying on the floor or bed

Notice the floor supporting you, as you take a gentle breath in, and notice the sounds in the room around you.

You might be able to hear distant sounds...

Listen gently to them as you become more aware of your breathing. Start to deepen your breath, right down to your tummy...

Filling your lungs with oxygen... and allowing the oxygen to spread through your body as you gently breathe out.

If you find your mind wandering during the meditation, just gently bring your attention back to your breathing. Acknowledge any thoughts that come to your mind, and trust that you will

recall them later, after the meditation, and gently let them go...
There is nowhere else you need to be right now... This is time
just for you... Feel your body becoming heavy against the floor,
as you start to relax...

We are going to give thanks to our body... our body works
tirelessly for us, day in and day out... and we don't always have
the time or energy to give back the nurturing and nourishment it
needs... so we will give our body gratitude now...

If any of your body parts are not working as you would
like... give them extra healing colour... and thank them for
trying... and perhaps promise to give them extra support...

As you breathe in now, imagine the air has a colour...
a soft, gentle colour... any colour that seems right for you...
breathe this colour in through the top of your head, your
crown... let it soak in through your hair... it is said that our
hair is our connection to our intuition... so thank your hair for
any guidance or insight it brings to you... thank your hair for
keeping your head warm... for helping you to look nice...

Feel the colour soak into your scalp, and inside your
mind... feel the colour sooth your brain, thanking it for always
working for you... for keeping you focused and intelligent... for
making sensible decisions and choices... allow your mind to rest
as you relax into this meditation...

Breathe the colour in through your eyes, bringing calm
to your eye lids... as they gently rest against your eye balls...
soothing them... thanking them for allowing you to see the
beauty in the world...

Breathe the colour in through your nose... thanking your
nose for allowing you to smell beautiful aromas and fragrances...
for keeping you safe... and in through your mouth... bringing
comfort to the back of your throat... relaxing your jaw, and your

teeth... letting go of any tension you may be holding there... giving thanks for all they do... assisting with your speech... and keeping you nourished...

Breathe the colour into your neck... your throat... down your trachea and your oesophagus... soothing your voice box... thanking your larynx for allowing you to speak your truth, quietly and with love...

Inhale deeply, bringing the colour into your lungs... opening the airways... breathing in health and healing... filling your blood with oxygen, and allowing your heart to send the healing colour around your body, with every beat... pulsating calmly... relaxed... give thanks to your heart and lungs for keeping you alive... for keeping your body fit and healthy...

Feel the colour surround your shoulders... around your chest and upper back... noticing any areas of tension... gently massaging them out... let the colour soak in to your shoulders... and spreading down the bone... relaxing the muscles that work for you tirelessly... down into your elbows... your forearm... let the colour fill your wrists with health... peace... relaxation... across the top of your hands... through the palms... thanking your hands for working continuously every day to grasp... lift... hold... for being flexible... feel the colour spread into your thumb... your second finger... your third finger... your ring finger... and fifth... give thanks ... both arms now heavy with relaxation...

Allow the colour to gently flow down your spine... gently stretching... aligning...relaxing... every vertebra happy... supported... and give thanks to each and every vertebra, disc, nerve and the fluid that runs through your spine... thank you for keeping you strong, supported, standing tall...

Breathe the colour into your tummy... calming your

digestive system... relaxed...peaceful... thanking it for keeping you healthy and nourished... allow the colour to flow... up to your chest... and down to your hips... feel your kidneys soften... gently supported... healthy...

Breathe the colour into your pelvis... relaxing your hips... your bottom... feel the colour seep into your bones... strong and healthy... relaxed... peaceful... give thanks for their strength... their support and stability... allow the colour to flow through your reproductive system... sending thanks for it functioning as it should in optimal health...

Allow the colour to flow into your hips... down your femur... relaxing these important muscles... always so strong and supportive... feel the colour surround your knees... bringing flexibility... calm... down your shin... your calf... and into your ankles... give thanks for their stability... lengthening the bones in your feet... comforting your heel... massaging along the sole of your foot... the arch... the ball of your foot... the colour flowing to your big toe... right to the tips of your nails... your second... third... fourth... and fifth toes... give thanks for their constant support... for keeping you grounded... both legs heavy... relaxed...

Notice any area in your body needing more relaxation... breathe your colour into this spot... breathing in healing... relaxation... calm... letting go any stress or tension with the out-breathe... continue with this for as long as you need...

Pause for as long as needed.

Gently bring your awareness back to the room now... become aware of your physical body... bring your awareness to your face... your neck... feel where your back touches the floor or chair... your hips... become aware of your arms and legs... gently wiggle your feet and hands... your ears... feel your body... solid and full of life...

Notice any sounds in the room around you... breathing in... feel your body physically present in this space... gently stretch and open your eyes when you are ready... keeping your gratitude for your body with you.

CHAPTER ONE
UNDERSTANDING YOUR CYCLE

"I empower myself with knowledge."

In an Australian study published in 2015, Kerry Hampton found that almost half of the women interviewed stated they knew when they ovulated. However, when they were tested, only 2.1% identified their ovulation date correctly. This means that often when a couple are trying to conceive, they are having intercourse at the wrong time of the month to get pregnant. By understanding how your body works, and by tracking your mucous for the cycle, you will know exactly the right times to have intercourse to optimise your chances for pregnancy.

Cycle apps are now very popular, but only provide feedback based on a normal cycle and the information you input, and do not consider a long or short luteal phase. While apps are a useful prompt to track your cycle, it is an unreliable method of obtaining pregnancy in most cases.

Even if you decide to see an IVF specialist, this information can be invaluable to your specialist for creating a plan for you and can make this process flow more smoothly. If you are single or same-sex and need to go to an IVF clinic for donor sperm, it can still be very beneficial to understand your cycle and give this information to your specialist.

Unfortunately, there is not an emphasis placed on education around women's bodies and how they work. There is an assumption that we are women, therefore we know. But in my experience, this simply isn't the case. I thought I had a good understanding. I'm female, I've had two children. I have PCOS. That qualifies me as an expert, yes? No. When I started working at the fertility clinic, I realised how much I didn't know about a cycle and how it actually works. Then I did my Natural Fertility Teacher Training and realised I still knew very little. How did I get to thirty-five years of age without understanding my menstrual cycle, something that was happening within my body every single month from when I was fifteen years old? My mum taught me the basics. I still remember those awkward yet profoundly inadequate and embarrassing sex lectures in high school, and I had read quite a bit when I was diagnosed with PCOS. So why did I still not know?

I firmly believe there is a fear that knowledge is power, and therefore a lack of knowledge keeps us 'behaving'. Don't tell them about sex and they won't do it. Well, guess what? They're going to do it anyway, so why not empower our daughters to understand their bodies so when they become sexually active, they already know when to avoid sex in order to *not* get pregnant, and when they are ready for a pregnancy, they can identify the right time of the month to try. I see so much fear, blame and guilt around people not getting pregnant when they are trying, and yet sometimes, it is as simple as they ovulate at a different time of the month, and they are not having sex then.

I believe we should have female-only menstruation education classes from ten years of age. Let's get educated before our first period so we know all about what that blood stain in our pants means—the first time it actually appears—so we are not scared, ashamed, or have any other variety of emotions it brings. I was lucky Mum had talked to me and my sisters about periods. When that moment arrived in a music lesson when I lay on the floor in the foetal position due to the horrific abdominal pain, only to discover the blood when I went to the bathroom, I knew exactly what it was. I remember walking home in such pain and went straight back to the bathroom. I called Mum in and asked, 'Is this what I think it is?' And she replied something along the lines of: 'Yep, welcome to being a woman.' It was normal, it was okay, I felt safe and aware despite in hindsight an incredible lack of knowledge. While my period was a really handy excuse to avoid swimming carnivals every year of high school, it would have been good if I'd understood it all a little more.

But what about the girls who don't have a mum or significant female in their life to teach them about these things. What about the girls whose mums don't understand and don't know how to teach their daughters, or don't want to. What about the women who still carry guilt and shame around becoming a woman, and therefore pass on that fear and judgement instead.

I would love to see government funded, women's health nurse run programs in schools from a young age. Let's remove the stigma, let's empower our young women through education and understanding, so they can make decisions appropriate for them.

My friend Jane knew I was doing my fertility teacher training, so she approached me when she was trying for her second baby. Her husband was away a lot for work, and they had been trying for several months with no success. She was starting to lose hope. I asked her if she understood what her mucous was telling her and she did *not*. We literally had a quick ten-minute chat about what it meant and when it meant she was fertile. The following month she was able to pinpoint exactly when she needed to have intercourse with her husband. This took the stress off both of them as finding the time around work and with a young child already at home was not easy. Limiting it to a few days instead of random, hurried moments over a whole month made the task more enjoyable and achievable. She got pregnant that month.

There is a lot of information out there and it can be overwhelming and confusing. For an in-depth and accurate explanation, please refer to the Billings Ovulation Method® by Evelyn Billings. Please don't believe everything you read on Dr Google, particularly well-intentioned but misinformed comments.

There is also no need to get your mucous between your fingers, stretch it, measure it, smell it or otherwise. Noticing the sensation of the mucous when you wipe is all you need to do, if the paper slips, you have slippery and therefore fertile mucous. One of the easiest ways to monitor your mucous is when you have a shower at night. Non-fertile mucous will wash away instantly. Fertile (slippery) mucous won't wash away immediately. The amount of mucous isn't important in determining the fertile window, so if you can recognise slippery and non-slippery mucous, you can generally identify ovulation.

The basics of a cycle is as follows:

The menstrual cycle begins with Day 1 of your bleeding, also known as a period, menstruation or menses, and continues until your next Day 1. This is normally 28-35 days in length and is usually quite regular. For some women however, it can be very irregular, ranging from days to months in length.

The menstrual cycle can be divided into four phases:

The Menstrual Phase

When a pregnancy does not occur in a cycle, the endometrium, or uterine lining, breaks down and results in a bleed. During menstruation, your oestrogen and progesterone levels are quite low, and your ovaries are fairly inactive. If you are doing blood tests to track your cycle, you would likely be told 'everything is baseline' during this time. We consider the first day of your period, your Day 1 of the cycle. Your period usually lasts around 4-7 days, but this will vary between each woman, and different ages. The cervix is open during menstruation, and as the bleeding diminishes, the cervix closes and a mucous plug forms within it.

The Follicular Phase

Unless you are having a short cycle, you will experience a variable time of infertility after your period (yes, some people do ovulate during their period), while the follicles within your ovaries begin to develop. The cervix is closed with a mucous plug during this phase, which protects the reproductive system from infection, and prevents sperm from entering. This stage will be dry with no mucous present, or some people experience a feeling of moistness with an unchanging type of mucous. Both of these are considered infertile. During the follicular phase, oestrogen levels rise, thickening the endometrium to prepare it for a pregnancy. Follicle Stimulating Hormone (FSH) also rises and assists to mature the eggs within the follicle. Generally, only one follicle will mature, but if more than one matures, this could result in a multiple pregnancy.

The Ovulation Phase

The developing follicles continue to produce oestrogen, activating the cervix to open and release the mucous plug, and produce the mucous essential for sperm survival. The presence of this mucous indicates fertility as this mucous nourishes and protects the sperm, maintaining their fertilising capacity for a few days, carrying the sperm through the cervix, the uterus and the fallopian tubes ready to connect with the ovulated egg. The pituitary gland triggers the release of a hormone called Luteinising Hormone (LH) which causes the mature follicle to burst, releasing the egg into a fallopian tube. When the egg leaves the follicle, the empty follicle becomes the corpus luteum, which produces oestrogen and progesterone, and continues to thicken the endometrium and nourish an embryo if it is made. The mucous in this phase changes from a moist to a wet to a slippery sensation. The last slippery day signifies ovulation most of the time. Progesterone starts to rise just before ovulation, causing the thickening of the mucous, which creates the noticeable change in mucous sensation. Pregnancy is possible on all days when fertile mucous is present and for 3 more days past ovulation (this allows for the lifetime of the egg and late ovulation, which can be 2 days after the last slippery day). The egg has a lifetime of 12-24 hours after it is released from the follicle, in which time it needs to be fertilised to result in a pregnancy.

Sperm can stay alive for up to four days when fertile mucous is present, so sex in the lead-up to ovulation day can still result in a pregnancy.

The Luteal Phase

The Luteal phase begins the day after ovulation until the start of your next bleed. If the egg is not fertilised, it disintegrates, causing the oestrogen and progesterone levels to drop. The endometrial lining breaks away and a period occurs. This phase is typically 14 days but can vary from 11-16 days in a normal cycle. A short luteal phase does not allow for an embryo to implant and results in an infertile cycle. This is usually caused by a drop in the hormones prematurely following an ovulation problem. A long luteal phase suggests pregnancy or incorrect identification of ovulation.

So, how does this information help you to become pregnant?

For pregnancy to occur, the following things must happen:
- The ovary must release a healthy egg into the fallopian tubes.
- Healthy sperm needs to be in the vagina when the fertile mucous is present.
- The fallopian tubes must allow the egg and sperm to travel unobstructed.
- If fertilisation takes place, the embryo must arrive within the uterus when the endometrium and embryo are at the right stage for implantation.

In addition to this, you:
- Must be able to identify your fertile mucous.
- Must have intercourse when there is fertile mucous present.

Have intercourse every second day during the slippery mucous phase if possible. A day off in between allows you to re-assess your mucous so you can identify ovulation. Have intercourse at other times during the month too, as you want to be replenishing the sperm, and also this allows you to have intercourse with your partner at times when there is no expectation of pregnancy occurring. This is important for a relationship, so neither party begins to feel 'used' or like a 'baby making factory'.

Journaling: reflection activity

1. Did you learn anything new about your cycle?
2. Is there information you knew or didn't know?
3. Does this change things for you now as far as when you are having sex, or giving you more control over when you are likely to be fertile?
4. Do you remember when you had your first period?

   How old were you?

   Did you know what it was?

   What were you feeling at the time?

   Did you have support?

   Are there any beliefs or experiences you are holding on to that you need to explore and process now?
5. What do you say about your period now? Is it painful and a nuisance or is it manageable? Explore the wording you use.
6. In your diary, start tracking your cycles. Write down the day your period starts, when it ends, when your slippery mucous starts and ends, when you believe ovulation to be, and how long between ovulation and your next period. This will give you so much information and will develop a connection with your body that you understand, and can support your body at the times it is needed. If you are trying for a baby right now, this could be the simplest thing you do to make that a reality.

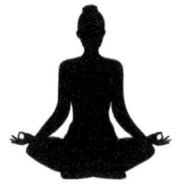

Meditation: for physical reproductive ailments

There is a lot of evidence to suggest the mind can have a great influence over the body and how it functions. This meditation focuses on clearing any reproductive system issues and bringing health and wellness to the reproductive system. There is a long relaxation in the beginning because this is vital to improving the effectiveness of the meditation and allowing the body to heal, so don't skip this part if it feels too long. Not all of the issues mentioned will apply to you, so if you're recording the meditation you might want to leave some parts out. This meditation is specific for women.

Just gently close your eyes. Take a few nice deep breaths. Just breathing in peace and starting to let go of any stress or tension that you feel within you. I want you to become aware of a vast space around you. A nice, dark, safe space. Surrounding your body. And as you open your eyes and look into this space, you notice in the distance a rainbow light. Full of blues, and greens, pinks, purples, orange, red and yellow... and any other beautiful, vibrant colours that you need right now.

As the light comes closer, notice it appears to be dancing... swirling around... carefree and happy. The light starts to surround you... swirling around your body... the energy of the light lifts your arms and legs, until you feel like you too are dancing with the light. The light has a strong energy... an uplifting and empowering energy. And as you dance with the light, it enters your body through your feet, and swirls up your legs and trunk, lifting you with its energy, as it flows down your arms, and up into your mind. The rainbow light exits out your fingertips, and out of your crown chakra, and your feet, until your whole body is glowing with these beautiful rainbow colours. Enjoy the feeling that this brings. The strong, positive vibes that this rainbow light brings to your body. Feel your body move freely, there's no restrictions of time or space, as you dance as one with the beautiful rainbow light.

When you are ready, your body returns to stillness, the rainbow light settles in front of you, and it circles in a ball. You reach out with your hands cupped... outstretched in front of you, and the rainbow light ball sits comfortably within your hands, as though it belongs there... as if it is part of you. And as you watch the ball, gently rotate in your hands, you feel the strength and the energy in your hands.

Become aware now of your reproductive system that would benefit from the healing energy you now have in your grasp. Feel in your body anywhere it is needed... it may be your ovaries, your fallopian tubes, your uterus... get a sense of which colour would best serve you at this time and see that colour coming out of the energy ball and into your fingers, though the palms of your hands and up your arms, and travelling to the part of your body where it is needed. See the colour starting in your ovaries... filling each ovary with healing light... gently healing any cysts... sending nourishing love filled light to your ovaries and the eggs within... when your ovaries feel healed allow the light to travel down each fallopian tube... clearing each tube as it moves through with flow and ease... gently dissolving any blockages you sense... as the healing light enters your uterus, allow it to spread throughout your womb… filling it with love… vitality… and health. See the lining thick, nourishing and welcoming to a future embryo… see the energy fill it with a vibrant, healthy colour…

Sit with the colour surrounding your whole reproductive system for a moment as it heals what is needed to be healed. As you relax and breathe, and let the colour do the job it has come here to do. It may be clearing blockages… calming overactive organs… or bringing life to those that need more vitality… you may need to bring in other colours or move it through to other parts of your reproductive system…

When the healing is complete, allow the colour to return back down your arms and out the palms of your hands or fingertips, back into the rainbow ball. And bring your attention to the rest your body and notice anywhere else that could benefit from the healing coloured light. Bring another colour from the ball through your fingertips or the palm of your hands, and up your arms, and take it to where it is needed in your body. Allow that colour to swirl round where it is needed. To fill that part of your body, to fill it with its healing energy, and to provide that part of your body with anything else that it might need… so that your whole body is connected and functioning as one…

When it is complete, allow that colour to again return down your arms, and out your hands and allow it to again join that swirling energy ball in your hands.

You might like to imagine storing this ball of energy inside of you somewhere for safe keeping… Or perhaps there is somewhere around you that you know you can keep it, so it will be there when you need it again. Find that place now, for your ball of energy…

And when it is safe, and you feel ready, just bring your awareness back now to your breathing. Become aware of where *your body meets the chair or floor. Feel the chair or floor hard beneath you, as you become aware of any sounds in the room... feel your body back in your physical body. You might lie to wiggle your fingers and toes. And when you are ready... take some nice deep breaths... and when you feel you are completely back in your physical body you can open your eyes.*

CHAPTER TWO
UNDERSTANDING INFERTILITY CAUSES

"There are many healthy changes I can make to help me have a baby."

So, what exactly is infertility? One scholarly article written by Zegers-Hochschild, defines infertility as, 'a disease of the reproductive system defined by the failure to achieve a clinical pregnancy after twelve months or more of regular unprotected sexual intercourse (et al., 2009, p4). And, at the time of writing this book, according to the Fertility Society of Australia's website, one in six Australian couples suffer infertility. This figure doesn't take into account the same-sex and single women that face infertility.

There are many physical causes for infertility. These include but are not limited to: Male issues such as no sperm, low sperm, poor quality sperm, a previous vasectomy or other structural issues. Female issues such as Polycystic Ovarian Syndrome (PCOS), endometriosis, structural or functional problems, age and weight. Lack of a vital component, such as single women or same-sex couples not having access to sperm. We will mostly focus on women's infertility; nevertheless, the notions are also for men.

There are many factors in our lives that can impact fertility.

Some of the most common causes are listed below with some healing guidance on how to begin aligning your emotional and physical ailments.

Stress and Anxiousness

I cannot emphasize enough the importance of managing your stress to promote a healthy, fertile cycle. You don't need to have much stress to affect your cycle. It could simply be the focus you are putting on trying to get pregnant—moving to a new house, a stressful day at work, illness or travel—any of life's stresses and daily duties can delay ovulation in your cycle. This is why it is vital to monitor your anxiety levels andj take simple steps to manage your stress. You might want to talk to a counsellor, start meditation, or simple techniques such as EFT. I will discuss stress in more detail later in the book.

Maintain a Healthy Weight

It is recommended that women maintain a body mass index (BMI) between 19-29 to maximize chances of conceiving, and for men a BMI below 29 is important for sperm health. Obese women, particularly those with central obesity, are less likely to conceive per cycle. Obese women often suffer menstrual cycle disturbance and are up to three times more likely to suffer oligo-/anovulation. A fine hormonal balance regulates follicular development and oocyte maturation, and obesity can alter this hormonal balance. Leptin is elevated in obese women and has been associated with impaired fertility. Obesity impairs ovulation but has also been observed to detrimentally affect endometrial development and implantation. The expression of polycystic ovary syndrome (PCOS) is regulated, in part, by weight, and so obese women with PCOS often experience more subfertility. Obesity also impairs the response of women to assisted conception treatments. Weight loss through lifestyle modification or other means has been demonstrated to restore a regular menstrual cycle and ovulation and therefore improve the likelihood of conception (Brewer & Balin, 2010).

Current research is showing obese men have more erectile dysfunction (ED) and low sperm counts. Overweight and obese men have been shown to have a 50% higher chance of encountering fertility problems compared to normal-weight men, and for every 3kg/m2 increase in the man's BMI, couples were 12% more likely to be unable to conceive. Serum testosterone levels were 25-32% lower in obese men than in normal-weight men, whereas oestrogen concentrations were 6% higher. Adipose tissue is an important site for hormone production; therefore, increased amounts of body fat lead to abnormal hormone regulation of testicular function (Bullen & Judge, 2015).

Weight management is best achieved through a healthy diet and regular exercise.

Diet

A healthy and nutrition rich diet is important for pregnancy. Talking to a dietician or nutritionist who is experienced in fertility could be very beneficial and provide you with support while you make healthy diet changes. In my experience, a Low GI diet or the Paleo diet have an incredible effect on the menstrual cycle, weight, general well-being and therefore fertility. Put simply, cutting out processed foods and increasing vegetable intake, will make a great difference to your health. Cutting out processed soft drinks or fruit juice and replacing it with filtered water is a very simple but effective change you can make to your diet. You may want to consider reducing caffeine intake or eliminating sugar and grains from your diet. Do not starve yourself, this will affect your menstrual cycle, as well as your mental and physical well-being. Plan your meals, have plenty of healthy vegetables in the fridge ready to go. Make healthy snacks you can grab when you are busy. Definitely do not go shopping hungry. Enjoy the process of finding new healthy recipes and creating nourishing meals, this is not only good for your body, but your mental health as well.

Exercise

Exercise does not have to be rigorous. A 30-minute walk each day is enough to start seeing weight loss, if needed. Overly-strenuous exercise has been found to be detrimental to fertility and hormone production, therefore a balanced and regular exercise program is recommended. Exercise is also good for your emotional well-being, which also improves your chances of conceiving. There are many books and DVDs available for Yoga and Fertility, and gentle exercises such as Tai Chi can have amazing benefits for your overall health and well-being. Joining an exercise class might be helpful in providing you support and a regular exercise regime.

Relationships

It is vital to *not* put trying to have a baby before the health of your relationship. When intercourse becomes a chore or purely for the goal of conception, and is no longer about intimacy between partners, this will lead to strain on your relationship and increased stress. Find ways to keep your relationship happy and loving. You might like to schedule a date night, or bond over healthy cooking or exercise together. Keep the process inclusive and keep the communication channels open. Intercourse at non-fertile times of the month takes the pressure off and helps you to connect on an intimate level that is not about making a baby. This is where tracking your mucous, and discussing your findings, is very beneficial to the health of your relationship.

Environmental Toxins

Toxins are synthetic chemicals that surround us in our everyday life. They fill our cleaning products, skin and hair care products such as soaps, moisturisers, baby wipes, perfumes. They are in our food and water supply, in the soil, sprayed directly on the food, and in the water intentionally or as a bi-product. They are put in our furniture, carpet, plastic containers, cookware and clothing. The plastic toys our kids play with, the pages of the books they chew on, the receipts from the shops we go to and every almost every single thing we touch.

Over 80,000 chemicals are used in every day products.

And we assume these products are safe because they are allowed in all of these products, but guess what? They are not regulated in this country, and therefore the safety of the chemical does not need to be proven before they go on the market. At the time of writing this there is no requirement to show these chemicals are safe before we are exposed to them. They are considered safe until proven otherwise.

And when it becomes apparent there is a link between a health issue and a chemical, the onus is on the person suggesting the link to prove the chemical is not safe (not the other way around) before it will be taken off the market. And when this is proven, as was the case with BPA, Bisphenol A (I am sure you have all seen BPA free plastic ware on the supermarket shelves), the company can simply replace the BPA with a different chemical and the cycle will need to start again.

BPA is found in plastic and the lining of cans (which then leaches into our food and water). Phthalates are in cosmetics, skin care and perfumes. Our food is sprayed with pesticides. All of our carpet, furniture, electronics and clothing, are filled with fire-retardants.

Many chemicals tested individually are deemed safe at the levels we are exposed to, but how often are we exposed to one single chemical at a time? Never. It's this compounding effect of different chemicals that is very difficult to measure and assess, but current research is showing some very concerning results.

I know this information is alarming, but don't be scared by it. Become empowered through research and be pro-active in making changes where you can.

Exposure to environmental toxins begins from the moment we are conceived. They cross the placenta and affect the development of the foetus.

At all other stages of life, they can enter our body via our:

1. Integumentary System (through the skin, what we touch or apply topically)
2. Digestive System (through our food, water, and medications/ supplements)
3. Respiratory System (what we breathe in)

The issue is, our endocrine system either mistakes these chemicals for hormones, or they interfere with our hormones, and create havoc in our bodies. For example, BPA mimics oestrogen. So, in pregnancy the placenta filters natural oestrogen and prevents it from crossing into the foetus. However, while BPA has endocrine and oestrogen activity, it is not recognised by the detoxification enzymes, and they pass freely through the placenta to the foetus.

New chemicals make it on to the market every day, and our defence mechanisms are not equipped to deal with them. We bombard our body every day with incessant and continuous exposure, and it is no wonder we are seeing a rise in infertility, cancers, auto-immune disorders, early puberty and many other health problems.

The issue seems completely overwhelming. Toxins are everywhere and in everything, so what can we possible do to stop it? The best thing you can do is minimise exposure wherever you can. Buy organic produce where you can. Buy fresh foods that haven't been exposed to packaging that leaches chemicals into our food and water. Invest in a good quality filter for your tap. Throw away your chemical filled self-care and cleaning products, and buy natural products, or make your own. Research furniture before you buy it, limit the plastic items that come into your house. There is so much you can do to reduce your exposure, so take the steps that are achievable and affordable for you. Start with the easiest and highest priorities and create other changes as you can. You don't need to do everything immediately. Educate your family and children, so they too can make better choices. People generally want to be healthy, and we trust the authorities to approve products that make this easy for us, but sadly it isn't the case, so we need to take our health and well-being into our own hands.

Smoking, alcohol or other drugs

Smoking/passive smoking and alcohol are proven to severely harm pregnancy, and lower sperm health. Some studies have found that women with a high alcohol intake take longer to become pregnant. The probability of conception in a menstrual cycle decreased with increasing alcohol intake in women, even among those drinking five or fewer drinks a week (Jensen et al, 1998). A study in Denmark between 1992 & 1994, found that female alcohol intake was associated with 2-3 times the adjusted risk of spontaneous abortion compared with no alcohol intake, and male alcohol intake was associated with 2-5 times the adjusted risk. Both male and female alcohol intakes during the week of conception increased the risk of early pregnancy loss (Jensen et al, 2004).

The result of a review of multiple studies, pointed towards a significant association between smoking and infertility with a 60% increase in the risk of infertility among cigarette smokers. There are also well-known negative effects of smoking on an eventual pregnancy and on neonatal well-being. Smoking is associated with an increased risk of miscarriage, bacterial vaginosis which is associated with late miscarriage, preterm labour, and with delivery of low-birthweight infants. Women attempting natural or assisted conception should be advised to stop smoking (Augood 1998).

Most of the reports showed that smoking reduces sperm production, sperm motility, sperm normal forms and sperm fertilising capacity through increased seminal oxidative stress and DNA damage. It is concluded that although some smokers may not experience reduced fertility, men with marginal semen quality can benefit from quitting smoking (Mostafa, 2009).

Age

Statistically, fertility begins to reduce from the age of 35, reducing significantly after age 40. From the age of 45-49 the likelihood is less than 5% and falls progressively to zero after this.

As you get older your cycles may become longer or more irregular, there are less fertile cycles, less mucous, and often shorter luteal phases. While there is nothing you can do to stop ageing, making the changes suggested above gives you the best chance of achieving pregnancy. If you are over 35 years old, you may want to discuss your options with a fertility specialist sooner rather than later.

Armed with this information, move on to the activities below. If you are feeling overwhelmed with information, give yourself the time you need to process or re-read as needed. Tracking your cycles can result in a pregnancy or can provide important information for your GP or Fertility Specialist if you need to progress further. Try not to get too stressed out about tracking—keep it as simple as possible—is it slippery or not? Make any changes to your diet and lifestyle that you can. Seek further help and investigations if they are needed.

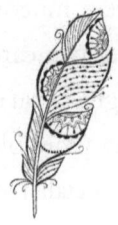

Journaling: fertility considerations

1. In your notebook, write down any reasons you are already aware of for your fertility issues. This may include lack of access to vital components, diagnosed medical conditions, physical issues, or any emotional reasons.
2. Do you have any of the issues outlined above?
3. Consider some other factors that perhaps could be affecting your fertility mentioned above. What changes can you make now to positively impact your fertility?

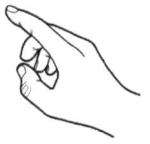

Tapping Script 1:
for fear you did something wrong

When faced with infertility, a natural response is to question if you have done something wrong to create the situation. You might start to analyse your eating habits, your previous sexual partners, your sleep patterns, if that bath was too hot that time. It would be a good idea to explore these ideas before you start tapping so you can make your tapping script specific to you. Everything I have written here are examples of things I have been told by people or things I experienced myself. But I want to make it very clear to you, this isn't your fault, you haven't done anything wrong. I have deliberately left this script generic, so you can make it unique to you, so please put your own words in where "*xxx*" is written.

Karate Point (KP): Even though I'm starting to wonder if this infertility is my fault,
I love and accept myself deeply and completely.
Karate Point: Even though I think I may have done something wrong to cause this,
I love and accept myself deeply and completely.
Karate Point: Even if I did something wrong,
I love and accept myself deeply and completely.
Inner Eyebrow (IE): I think this might be my fault

Outer Eye (OU): I think I caused it

Under Eye (UE): oh no, did I do this?

Under Nose (UN): did my behaviour make this happen?

Under Mouth (UM): is it because I thought "*xxx*"?

Collarbone (CB) *use fist*: or because I did "*xxx*"?

Under Arm (UA) *use hand*: I always knew I would pay for that one day

Top of the Head (TH): that karma would come around

IE: I haven't always had the best diet

OE: I eat too much "xxx"

UE: sometimes I drink too much

UN: there were a few times I drank way too much

UM: did that cause this?

CB: there was that time I did "xxx"

UA: did that cause this?

TH: is this really my fault?

IE: I haven't always made the best choices

OE: with my health

UE: with my partners

UN: I haven't always been as nice as I could have been

UM: sometimes my emotions run away from me

CB: is this payback?

UA: is this karma?

TH: is this all my fault?

Keep going as long as you need to,

being as specific to your circumstances and feelings as you can be.

IE: logically I know this isn't my fault

OE: but the fear remains

UE: I want to let it go

UN: I know this belief isn't helping me

UM: the fear keeps me stuck

CB: the guilt keeps me trapped

UA: it's time to let it go

TH: once and for all

IE: so, I am choosing to forgive myself

OE: for anything I did wrong

UE: for anything that may have contributed to this infertility

UN: I am choosing to love myself

UM: just as I am

CB: I am choosing to forgive myself

UA: for anything I may have done wrong

TH: and I am choosing to let this fear and guilt go

IE: it doesn't serve me any purpose

OE: other than keeping me stuck

UE: and I am choosing to not remain here

UN: I am freeing myself

UM: I am letting myself off the hook

CB: so I can move forward

UA: I forgive myself

TH: <u>this isn't my fault.</u>

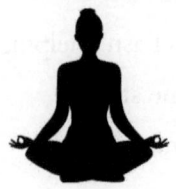

Meditation: for improving health

This meditation also has a long relaxation stage. Relaxing the body is vital for good health, and the deeper you can go into meditation the more effective it will be in creating long-lasting changes for you. Relaxation is key to a deep level of meditation. This meditation focuses on letting go of unhealthy patterns and behaviours and encouraging healthier lifestyle changes. This meditation is suitable for both men and women.

Find a comfortable position. You might like to sit in a chair with your feet firmly planted on the floor. Or you might like to lie down with a pillow and a blanket. Gently close your eyes and set the intention to take this time for healing...

Once you are comfortable, bring your attention to your breathing. Notice the breath coming in, and gently letting it out. You might like to deepen your breathing slightly, taking a deep, long, slow breath in to the bottom of your tummy, and gently let it turn and release it.

Begin to notice any stress or tension starting to leave with the out breath. Continue to breathe this way for a few moments. Just noticing your body starting to feel heavy against the floor or the chair... as you become aware of where your body meets the floor or the chair. Along your back, your bottom, your feet, allow them to sink in... notice any thoughts that come to you as you relax, and let them go...

Now notice the sensation of safe, comforting hands placed gently on your head. And where those hands meet your head, just feel the sensation of relaxing spread across your scalp, and down around your face. Feel your eyes gently closed and relaxed, not needing to see anything external at this time. Allow the relaxation to extend to your nose, along your cheek bones, as your face gently relaxes. Allow your mouth to relax now, there's nothing it needs to say or do right now. This is time just for you, just to be, just to relax...

Allow the sensation of relaxation to spread down over your ears, down over your neck. Just allow your neck to relax now and soften. Feel those comforting hands rest gently on both shoulders. Feeling the sensation of the relaxation extending across your shoulders, massaging in between your shoulder blades, allowing any tension... any knots... to start releasing. Feel the relaxation spread gently down your spine, relaxing... lengthening every vertebra, and allow the sensation to spread out to your ribs, become aware of the extension between your ribs as you breathe in... and as you gently breathe out let it relax, feeling any stress starting to go.

Allow the relaxation to spread around to the front of your chest, down both arms like a gentle massage... going over those muscles in the tops of your arms, down into your elbows, your lower arms... relaxing your wrists and all the bones in your hands, feeling each finger lengthening and relaxing.

Allow the sensation of relaxation to run down both your sides and across your tummy. Allow yourself to sink heavily... as you relax deeper and deeper into the meditation.

You might like to feel the hands go gently down your back and rest at your lower back, removing any stress or tension that you are holding there, and feel the relaxation spread from your lower back into your hips... your pelvis... into the tops of your legs that are busy holding us up all day long... now is the time to let them relax. Feel this calmness stretch further down into your legs, through your knees and down into your lower legs. Relax your ankles, both of your feet... imagine the relaxing hands holding both of your feet... as you feel where they connect to the floor. Feel them extend from here down through the floor, into the earth. Keeping your body safe and grounded for this meditation.

Now in your mind's eye see yourself standing in your home... notice how you look... if you're healthy... notice your weight without judgement, but simply awareness... as if watching yourself in a movie, see yourself move throughout your day... notice what you eat... if you exercise... any unhealthy habits you may have that you no longer want. See yourself go to work, or any other daily practices you attend to... are those things helpful to your fertility journey? Notice if they make you happy... healthy... As you watch yourself now, without judgement, notice one thing you would like to change to create a happier and healthier you... it might be eating better... it might be exercising... it might be letting go of unhealthy habits... now see yourself start to do this as your movie plays out in front of you... see yourself making that healthy change... see how your body becomes more vibrant and healthy as you make this change... see a glow around your reproductive system as it becomes healthier... better functioning... grateful for the changes you are making... see the people in your life supporting you... noticing the healthy changes and the difference in you... see yourself looking vibrant... healthy... happy... forgive yourself for any past habits or behaviours you had that weren't healthy... and send encouragement and love to yourself now for making healthy and long-lasting changes... spend a few moments now enjoying this feeling…

Bring this feeling back with you now, knowing this feeling is always within you… as you start to notice your breath once more… notice where your body meets the floor or the chair. Feel your body… your back, or your bottom or your feet touch the floor or the chair. And bring your awareness back into these body parts. As you breathe in feel your physical body start to awaken. Notice where your feet meet the floor and start to give them a little wiggle… bringing full sensation back into your feet and the rest of your body. Take some nice deep breaths in and let them out… allow yourself to feel present in your physical body and in the room around you. Continue to wiggle your toes… your fingers… and allow movement into the rest of your body. When you are ready you can open your eyes. You might like to stay sitting there for a moment, just recalling any guidance or insight that you received. And when you are ready, you can feel refreshed and rejuvenated, ready for the day…

CHAPTER THREE
TUNING IN TO YOUR EMOTIONS

"It is safe to feel my emotions and to listen to what they are telling me."

What if I was to challenge your story?

I don't intend for this to sound confronting although, I'm aware it might, so please bear with me. Sometimes our beliefs are so ingrained we don't ever question them, but if we can learn to, we can make great changes in our life. So please read on with an open mind and see where it takes you.

What if I told you that it doesn't matter that your mum has endometriosis, that just because all your sisters have PCOS doesn't mean you have it too, that just because all of your friends needed IVF doesn't actually have any bearing or influence on your fertility and chances of successful pregnancies? What if I stood in front of you right now and asked you to change the script and let that story go—to redefine who you are and your fertility story—would you be angry at me? Indignant? Perhaps say, 'Who the hell do you think you are? I know my story! It's my story and I'm keeping it.'

But what if you just took a moment to let go of the anger and the need to own it? What if you *questioned* your story? What is it that makes you so readily accept that story as your own? Why are you so eager to keep it and how does it serve you? Why don't you want to change your story, or better yet, let it go completely?

Here's an even more confronting question: If I asked you right now to let that story go forever, to never re-tell it to another person, to stop believing it, would you do it? Would you be prepared to exchange your story for the baby you so desperately want?

It's time to question your story.

A lot of our value systems and the beliefs we hold are not actually ours. They are inherited or learned from our parents, our grandparents, our teachers, friends and colleagues. We may have watched a movie or documentary that had a specific belief system or read a book that we accepted as fact. As children we are generally not encouraged to question the *facts* or the authority figures that teach them. To do so is seen as disruptive and difficult. To be the *good* child we accept what we are told, and we behave accordingly. This can easily transfer into adulthood. Questioning those who are *superior* to us can feel very uncomfortable especially if it is not something you have previously done. Perhaps it simply doesn't occur to you to question what you are told. If that's the case, it's about to change. This book will ask you to question everything. What you've been told, what you've learnt, what you have believed to be true. This doesn't mean you go out and confront everyone that's ever told you a false truth (even if it was well meaning). This is very much a personal journey and is about your growth, healing, and journey, towards becoming a parent. If you find yourself blaming and getting angry at others, please write it down in your journal as you read through these pages, but try to refrain from having it out with other people until you have done your work and processed how you actually feel about the situation—fully. This book will ask you to explore all of these beliefs and where they came from. And, it will also ask you to take responsibility for your life and your circumstances. Looking to blame others will hold you back from the healing process.

Depending on what you have believed to be true throughout your life about your ability to have children, could be affecting your current situation.

For example, a client stated, 'I only have to look at a guy and I'm pregnant.' This statement was followed by, 'My mum was the same.' Indeed, she did get pregnant very easily. In some ways, this belief is as harmful as thinking that you *can't* have children. There is a fear that goes along with every sexual encounter, if you believe it, it may result in an unwanted pregnancy.

Another client said her mother had terrible pregnancies and issues with endometriosis; however, she always told her children that her story was not theirs, and there was no reason to believe they would suffer the same fate. Despite my client having endometriosis, she got pregnant easily and has not suffered in the same way her mother did. Her mother gave her a gift by being positive and encouraging despite her experiences. My client always believed she would not suffer the same fate as her mother because she was told she would not.

The same can be said for believing you can't have children. I know when the doctor told me I had to have my children before I turned 28, I believed it. And certainly, after I hit this age, my periods became more and more irregular, and I never became pregnant again.

Another client told me she knew she would have trouble having children—because her mother did, and her grandmother did, and it was in her genes. Not surprisingly, she did have a lot of trouble getting pregnant, and had to clear a lot of issues and beliefs that were inherited in order to conceive.

Interestingly, I have spoken to many women who are shocked to discover their infertility when they start trying to have children later in life. Some were never told it might be difficult, or never held a belief one way or another. However, sometimes women tell me that other people warned them that if they put their career first, they would not have children, or if they didn't find Mr Right soon and marry, they would not have children, or if they are single or same-sex they were giving up their right to have children. Even though these beliefs were not their own, it still affected them. It was when the infertility diagnosis was put on the table that they started to wonder. Were they right? Is this true? Was I selfish or silly or naïve to think I could have a career and a baby, or love another woman and have a baby, or have a baby on my own or whatever the situation is? Once the seed of doubt is planted, the belief takes hold. Identifying where these beliefs come from, recognising them as your own or inherited, and letting them go goes a long way in the emotional ability to conceive a child.

You will likely find as you begin your infertility journey that everyone will start to offer advice and opinions. Usually people are trying to be helpful and sometimes it is, but often it's not. If, however someone makes a comment that hits a nerve or has you questioning yourself, it's worth exploring this further. Why does it resonate with you? Ask yourself why you can let some comments go without giving them a second thought and yet this one has stayed with you? Is there an element of truth in it, is there a change you need to make or are you holding onto a false belief about some aspect of it that you need to process and let go of?

Addressing these beliefs early in the journey will also help in not owning any guilt or blame as the process unfolds. Emotions and infertility are complicated enough without taking on other people's beliefs and judgements as your own.

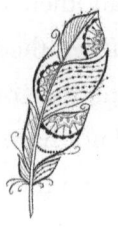

Journaling: embrace your emotional self

In your workbook, consider these questions:

1. How many children did your mum, grandma, aunty and sister have? What stories have they told about it? Was it easy or difficult? Have you repeated these stories throughout your life? How does this relate to your current situation?
2. Do your friends have children? Have they had fertility issues? What have they told you about it? Does this affect you in any way?
3. What are *your* beliefs on your current situation with regards to finances, career, living situation, relationship etc?
4. What are the beliefs of *those around you* on your current situation with regards to finances, career, living situation, relationship etc?
5. Write a list of all the beliefs you can think of that you have around fertility. Now go through this list and mark off the ones you feel are your beliefs, or if not, who they belong to. Can you consider there might be a different way of looking at it?
6. Next to each point on the list, write a new affirmation that accepts your current situation. Here are some affirmations for you to use, or make up your own:

Belief: "All the women in my family have trouble getting pregnant, it's in our genes."

Affirmation: "I choose to create a new story for me, where I am fertile and become pregnant easily."

Belief: "I am in a same-sex relationship, and my friend casually told me I had chosen not to have children because of this, maybe she is right."

Affirmation: "Regardless of who I love, it is my birthright as a woman to be a mother, and my child will be loved and cared for."

Belief: "I am single, so if I have a baby on my own, people will think I had a one-night stand."

Affirmation: "I am a strong and independent woman, who is more than capable of being a single-mum, and no-one but me needs to know my story."

7. If any of your new affirmations don't feel 'true' to you, then you will need to do some more work on these to clear the beliefs. It would be helpful to write your affirmations down and place them somewhere you will see them every day, on the bathroom mirror is a great place for this. Repeat them to yourself morning and night.

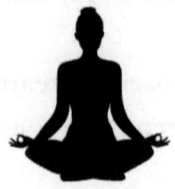

Meditation: for motherhood

This is a general meditation for seeing beyond infertility, to being pregnant and or being a mum. Often when the focus is only on getting pregnant, we don't consider how life will be after this point, and it can come as a big shock when we are pregnant or when we are a mum. This meditation is most suitable for women.

Find a place to sit where you are comfortable, and your back is supported. You might like a blanket to keep you warm. Take a deep breath in, down to your toes and gently let it go. As you breathe in, fill your body with peace, and as you breathe out, start to release any tension you are holding in your body... Becoming aware of your body as it presses against the chair or the floor. Notice your whole body, relaxing any areas of tension with every breath in...

Visualise a healing white light, entering your body from the tip of your head. Feel it light up your mind, your eyes, your ears, your nose, your mouth. Feel the light glide down the back of your head and around to your jaw. Let your jaw relax, and rest comfortably. Feel the light carry this relaxation down to your neck and across your shoulders and chest and upper back. The light flows down both arms, past your elbows, and into your hands and to the tips of your fingers. As the light fills your trunk, let it light up your heart, your lungs, your tummy, and your lower back. Feel the tension lift as the light travels down to your pelvis, through your hips, your knees, your calves and into your ankles and feet and toes. Feel your whole body relax now it is filled with this healing white light.

In your mind's eye, see yourself sitting comfortably as you look towards your stomach… you notice a baby bump… notice how this makes you feel… allow any emotions to come and sit with this as long as you need to… knowing your baby is safe within your belly… you might like to place our hands across your tummy as you connect with the baby within…

When you are ready move forward in time and see a much bigger tummy… you can feel your baby kicking now… again notice any feelings or emotions that come up for you… notice the people around you… those who are there to support you in this journey… see their smiling faces… see how loved you and your unborn baby are…

Again when you are ready move forward to the delivery of your baby… notice who is there to support you… a loved one, family or friends… the helpful doctor or midwife… everyone is supporting you and your baby as it arrives safely into the world… see yourself holding your baby for the first time… look in to your babies eyes… you might be aware if your baby is a boy or a girl… you may even have a name chosen already… enjoy this time holding your beautiful healthy baby for as long as you like…

Moving forward in time when you are ready, see yourself at home, looking after your baby… notice how you look and feel without any judgement, send love to yourself for the great job you are doing… notice who is around to support you… see the beautiful connection you share with your child as you watch your baby grow into a toddler…

Spend as much time as you need to in this moment… notice

any feelings or fears that may come to you... fill them with love and let them go... know you are safe, you are strong, you are a very good Mum.

When you are ready, start to notice the sounds around you, in the room where you are sitting, as you begin to settle comfortably back into your physical body. Become aware of your body and where your body meets the chair or floor. Become aware of your breathing, as you gently wake. Take some nice deep breaths in, and when you are ready, you can gently open your eyes, and sit still for a few moments, soaking in the feelings you experienced in this meditation. You may like to journal these thoughts and feelings, or any insights that came to you. If you experienced any fears or uncomfortable feelings, journal these to work through later.

CHAPTER FOUR
HOW FEELINGS EFFECT FERTILITY

"I acknowledge and respect my feelings as I work through them."

Usually when you start thinking about having a baby, you begin to notice babies everywhere. You smile at them and feel that stirring in the pit of your stomach, where you plan to have a baby of your own someday soon. All of your friends start having babies and you love to visit and buy them things, imagining that time in the not too distant future when you will be shopping for your own baby.

Nonetheless, time goes on ... and you don't become pregnant. And, all of a sudden, those babies you see everywhere, and your happy mum-friends become a painful reminder of what you do *not* have, and what you may never have. You stop visiting your friends and their babies because it simply hurts too much. You stop shopping in the baby section of the shops because every dummy or triple-zero jumpsuit is like a knife stabbing you directly through the heart.

You no longer smile at the babies down the street and instead look at them with distaste. You eye the parents resentfully, perhaps judging their ability to be a good parent, knowing you could do it so much better if only given the chance.

You might start to blame God or some Higher Power, for punishing you by withholding the one thing you desperately want.

Sex is no longer a beautiful connection between you and your partner, but an angry chore that ultimately will fail you.

You might blame your body for not doing what it is meant to do. You might call it names such as stupid or useless. You may begin to actually hate your body and stop taking appropriate care of it.

You become angry, bitter and resentful. You are hurt. You are hurting.

And this is okay... for a while. The problem a lot of people encounter is they unpack and live here. The anger and emotions become who they are and their story which makes it very difficult if not impossible to move forward.

Don't get me wrong, it's very important to acknowledge your feelings. You need to be heard and understood, and you can do this for yourself. You don't need validation from anyone else that how you are feeling is right or wrong. You certainly don't need anyone else to come in and 'fix' you. You have the power within you to take care of you and give you what you need.

But ask yourself this: 'If I look at every baby I see with distaste, if I look at every parent I see with anger, resentment or hate, if I cannot look at anything loosely related to having a baby because it makes me so sick to my stomach, what am I telling the Universe? That I want a baby or that I do not?'

There are many Universal Laws that come into play here. What we put out is what we get back. What we wish for others we receive in return. The Law of Attraction, the Law of Gratitude, trusting in Universal powers and Divine Timing. And usually a whole lot of emotional and spiritual growth. However, it's all well and good to know this logically, but have you ever tried to switch a feeling off? Everyone has experienced irrational anger they can't explain, jealousy they want to pretend is not there, getting over a lost love you desperately still want to be with. Humans are emotional beings.

That's what makes us human. When your feelings start to dictate your thoughts and behaviour though it can lead to problems.

Notice where or who you direct your emotions at. Are you holding them all in and hurting yourself or are you letting them explode out towards others? Usually we let them out at the people we love the most, your significant other, your parents, siblings, friends. This can very quickly lead to a breakdown in relationships and the loss of friendships. If you become short tempered at work, it won't take long to get the unwanted attention of your colleagues and employers. If you start looking for people to blame you could easily hurt those closest to you such as your parents or partner. Chances are you don't even believe what you're saying but you're hurting, and you need to get it out.

Keep working through this book and you will be armed with tools that are practical and effective, rather than lashing out and making an already difficult situation even harder.

Our feelings often present physically in our bodies. Identifying this can help to process it and manage it instead of it controlling us. Consider the emotions you are currently feeling around your infertility. What's the first one that comes to mind? Anger is a very common feeling when experiencing infertility. Journaling your anger and who it is directed at can give you very helpful information for the tapping exercises provided in this book. Another way to make tapping even more effective is noticing where your feelings are located in your physical body. Sit with your anger for a moment then do a mental scan of your body. Where is it located? Anger often presents as a 'fire in your belly'. You might find your arms are tense, your fists clenched. Your jaw and neck could be tight with your shoulders held up, eyes narrowed. Your body is ready to fight. Write all of this down in your journal to tap on. Now breathe and let go of all the tension you are holding onto.

Sadness is also a common emotion. Sit with your sadness. Where is it? Often, it's an ache in our chest, a heavy heart. Tears might fill our eyes; our body could feel deflated like there's no strength left to hold us up. Become aware of your body and how the sadness is expressing itself physically and write all of this down. Now take a deep breath and let it go for the time being.

Fear is a huge emotion, although perhaps not one we recognise a lot in infertility. Fear of the unknown, fear of never being a parent, fear our partner might leave if we can't provide the family they want, fear you will go bankrupt trying to make it happen. Fear you will never be quite fulfilled in life, always waiting, always hoping for more. Sit with fear for a moment, recognise your fears and name them in your journal. Where do you feel fear in your body? Does your heart race? Does your throat tighten? Are you holding your breath? Notice it, write it all down, then take a deep breath and let it go.

Before you move on to the activities, I want you to experience a happy emotion, so you can recognise the difference in your body. Imagine holding the baby you love in your arms, knowing everything is perfect. Your baby is healthy, you are healthy, your partner if you have one is happy, everything is good, you are safe to feel happy. Where is happiness in your body? You probably have a smile on your face. You might have tears in your eyes, but this will feel different to the tears of sadness. You will likely feel a warmth in your chest, your heart beating slow, steady and strong. Your arms and legs will most probably feel relaxed and free. You might feel a lightness you haven't felt for a while, like you can breathe again, the weight of the world that was on your shoulders now gone. This is the feeling you want to aim for when doing your healing work. Recreating how you will feel holding your newborn baby is the goal of using affirmations and doing your tapping.

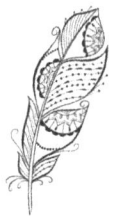

Journaling: clearing emotions by clearing the mind

Allow yourself an hour for this activity where you will not be interrupted. Get your workbook and sit where you are comfortable. Ask yourself the following questions and answer them as honestly as you can. Write as much as you need to so that you feel you have 'got it all out'. Write in the way you feel, use childish language, swear words, be resentful, bitter, angry, hurt—whatever you are feeling is what you are feeling—and that is okay. This activity is for you, and no one else.

Think back to the first time you imagined being a mum. How did you feel? What did you imagine it would be like? How many children did you plan to have? Were they boys or girls? Did you name them? Did you imagine being in a relationship? What was that like? How did you imagine your pregnancy to be? What was the labour like in your imagination? Had you thought of these things? What was the future of your children like? Did you see them growing up? Going through school? Graduation? Careers? Husbands/wives/children of their own? Write it all down, every last detail.

Enjoy this feeling for a while, knowing it is still within reach.

Now think about the first time you thought you could be pregnant and found out you were not. This may not have happened yet, happened only once or many, many times. Write about these and how it made you feel.

Pay particular attention to: How you feel about seeing other people with children, what your thoughts and opinions are of them. How have these changed from your original opinions?

How you react to baby clothes or baby products in shops. Who do you blame for not being pregnant? Yourself, your partner, God, your body, someone or something else? Write all of this down, in as much detail as you can.

Sit with these emotions for a while, know it is okay to feel all of this. Cry if you need to, scream, shout, hit a pillow. Just get it out of your body!

Now go through everything you have written and highlight the important parts. The words or feelings you can see that are not conducive to getting pregnant and welcoming a baby into your body or life.

Draw a table with two columns, and in dot points write in the left column all of the words or statements you have highlighted.

Now next to these, write new beliefs. Note if these don't feel 'true' to you, you can start them with "I choose to feel…" as this may be easier for your body to believe, plus it gives you some power back over your feelings.

Read over these new statements every morning and night. Cross them out once you no longer feel you need them. Add to them when something new arises. Change the wording as your experience and beliefs change. Remove the 'I choose to…" when you start to really believe the statements.

Be aware of your feelings around babies and parents and repeat the exercise as often as you need to. Some days will be easier and some harder, but know it is all part of your journey and it is okay, so long as you are doing something about it.

Some examples for you to use:

Feeling: "I feel like my heart is breaking every time I see baby food at the supermarket."

Affirmation: "I choose to look at the baby food and imagine which ones my future children will enjoy."

Feeling: "I hate this useless body for not being able to get pregnant."

Affirmation: "I keep my body strong and healthy with good food and exercise and thank it for the baby it will one day carry."

Feeling: "My friends get pregnant at the drop of a hat and they don't even appreciate it!"

Affirmation: "I don't know anyone else's story, but I am happy for my friends when they have babies, and trust that my turn is coming soon."

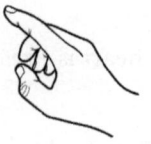

Tapping Script 2:
for jealousy of other people having babies

This is a really difficult one, especially when it's your closest friends or family that are having the babies. It is easy to fall into the trap of feeling resentment, anger and jealousy. Often this leads to you also feeling a whole lot of guilt for having those feelings. You end up with a cocktail of emotions swirling around, changing from one second to the next and leaving you completely overwhelmed and upset. Remember it's okay to feel these things, but you want to put the time and effort in to processing them and working through them instead of taking it out on the people you love around you. It's not always easy but try to remember how you would want them to react if you announced you were the one having a baby and they were still infertile.

Karate chop (KP): Even though I feel jealous of those around me,
I love and accept myself deeply and completely.
Karate chop: Even though I'm struggling to feel happy for others,
I love and accept myself deeply and completely.
Karate chop: Even though I'm so angry right now,
I love and accept myself deeply and completely.

Inner eyebrow (IE): It's so unfair

Outer Eye (OE): why do they get to have babies when I don't?

Under Eye (UE): are they more deserving than me?

Under Nose (UN): look at them flaunting their big tummies

Under mouth (UM): it makes me so angry

Collarbone (CB) *use fist*: I am so angry

Under Arm (UA) *use hand*: all of this anger in my body

Top of the head (TH): I feel like I might explode

IE: going to these baby showers

OE: it's killing me

UE: pretending to be happy

UN: when I just want to scream

UM: why them?

CB: why not me?

UA: what did I do wrong?

TH: I can't take much more

IE: I know it's not their fault

OE: but this hurts so much

UE: that's why I hold on to my anger so tightly

UN: because otherwise I will just feel sad

UM: and that sadness might kill me

CB: I can't take the sadness

UA: it feels like giving up

TH: at least with anger there's still a chance

IE: I'm still fighting for it

OE: I don't want to give up

UE: but it's so painful to keep wanting

UN: and to keep going without

UM: and I'm constantly being reminded

CB: by everyone around me

UA: baby showers

TH: talking about their kids in the lunch room

IE: I don't want to know

OE: can't they see they're hurting me?

UE: every time they mention their pregnancies

UN: or their children

UM: I hate it

CB: I hate feeling this way

UA: I feel so much guilt for feeling jealous

TH: I don't want to feel like this anymore

Keep going as long as you need to, being as specific to your circumstances and feelings as you can be.

IE: I need to start taking care of me

OE: all of this anger and hurt isn't helping me

UE: it doesn't help my body to have a baby

UN: I don't want to be this person anymore

UM: I want to be supportive of my friends

CB: but I can choose to not be around it all the time

UA: I can say no when I'm not feeling strong enough

TH: I give myself permission to take care of me first

IE: my friends will understand

OE: and if they don't that's still okay

UE: because my health is important

UN: and I am the only one that can look after it

UM: so, I am choosing to put me first

CB: and when I'm feeling good

UA: and strong

TH: I can be around my friends and their babies

IE: I have tools I can use

OE: I can tap before I see them

UE: I can journal how I'm feeling

UN: I can process the guilt rather than let it consume me

UM: I can feel the anger then let it go

CB: I can feel the hurt because I'm hurting

UA: I give myself permission to feel all of these things

TH: but I trust that I will be okay.

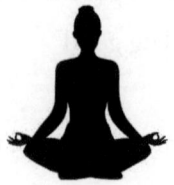

Meditation: for feeling joy when you see a baby

When we have been trying for a baby for some time and not getting pregnant, it can become very difficult to see other people with their babies, or to pass through the baby section of a store. This meditation focuses on recognising those emotions and helping to clear them, so you can find joy in spending time with other people and their children. This meditation is suitable for men and women.

Find yourself in a comfortable position. Allow your body to relax into the chair. Soften your shoulders... Have your feet sitting firmly on the ground, keeping you strong but comfortable. Become aware of any sounds around you within the room... Any smells you might notice... allowing them to bring you comfort in this journey. Take your awareness further outside of your room now... and become aware of any sounds outside... Perhaps there's traffic or birds... let the sounds just drift off into the distance as you bring your attention to your body.

Now feel a white light travel down over your head... bringing with it peace and love and relaxation. Feel it going across your eyes as you let them relax... comfortable and peaceful. Down over your nose and across your cheek bones. Feel the white light relax your jaw and your mouth... It doesn't need to do any work at the moment, and it can take this time just to relax and re-energise. Feel the white light to travel down over the top of your head and the back of your head… into your neck. Relaxing your ears… they only need to concentrate on my voice for this time, everything else can wait.

Allow your throat to soften… there's nothing you need to be able to say right now. Feel the white light go into your back, between your shoulder blades… massaging out any tension that might be held there. Feel the white light travel across your chest… into your shoulders, relaxing the joints. Down through the muscles of your arms, past your elbows… and down into your wrists and your hands. Let your arms feel heavy, as your hands gently rest in your lap or down by your sides. Allow the white light to relax the trunk of your body as it gently drifts around you, down through your back… relaxing your spine. Feeling it straighten and then soften gently against the chair or floor.

Let your tummy relax… and if you are holding any knots or tension there, allow it to start to dissolve as your body becomes heavier. Breathe down into your body, deep into your tummy… bringing oxygen into your tummy through the white light, so that it can relax.

Bring the white light down through your legs, through your knees… as they feel heavy against the chair or floor. Take a deep breath, bringing oxygen all the way down to your feet, and into your toes. Just notice if there are any other areas of tension in your body that need to be relaxed for this meditation and bring the white light to those areas. Breathe in oxygen to those body parts that need it now… allowing your body to feel heavy, relaxed and peaceful.

Now in your mind's eye see yourself sitting in a quiet shopping centre… it's early and no-one else is there yet as you wait for the shop to open… as you sit there notice any thoughts that come, acknowledge them and let them go… as you sit there a lady begins to walk towards you with a baby in a pram... notice how this sight makes you feel... there's no judgement here, just simply allow the feelings to come... there's no right way to feel... just feel... allow your emotions to flow freely... let them out... send love to yourself at this time... and if it feels okay to do so, send love to the lady and her baby... knowing your time will soon come and the love you send out in to the world will flow back to you also... the lady and her baby have left now and you are sitting alone again... again notice how you are feeling and allow any emotions to surface...

When you are ready you see the shop open and you make your way inside... you find your way to the baby section... you see tiny little outfits, dummies, nappies... again allow yourself to feel anything that comes now without judgement... send love to yourself... there's no-one else around so let your emotions flow freely... this is a safe place for you to feel anything you are feeling... you might like to pick a jumpsuit up... feel the fabric in your hands... as you do so you feel a knowing within you that one day your baby will wear this jumpsuit... you can enjoy this moment if it feels safe to do so... feel the weight and the warmth of a baby in your hands now... notice how this feels... send love to yourself and to the baby and to the jumpsuit and all of the other items in the baby section of the store... it is safe to want these things... it is okay to feel any emotions you are now feeling... savour the feeling of holding that baby... spend a few moments now enjoying this feeling...

When you are ready, carry this feeling with you as you leave the store... knowing at any time when you are feeling sad you can re-visit this feeling to remind yourself of the possibilities... the deep knowing within you... breathe a deep breath down into your lungs, as you become aware again of the sounds outside of the room... gently bring them back into your focus, and then start to acknowledge the sounds in the room around you. Notice if it is warm or cool... become aware of where your body is meeting the chair or floor... of where your feet are resting on the floor. And breathe life back into your physical body... allow some gentle movement into your hands and feet. You might like to wiggle your hands and feet, your mouth. And when you are ready you can open your eyes.

CHAPTER FIVE
BELIEFS ON YOUR ABILITY
TO BE A PARENT

"I can choose to be the parent I want to be."

Very often we desperately want children but have an underlying belief that we will not be any good at it. There are so many reasons for this, but I will explore some of the most common I have come across here. It's important to note that these beliefs affect both parents, and for best results, both parents need to address any issues they hold around this.

'I am too selfish to be a parent.'

I have heard this often from friends. They either really believe they are too selfish or have been told by someone else (often their mother) that they are too selfish to have children. Firstly, being 'selfish' isn't necessarily a bad thing. There is absolutely nothing wrong with taking care of our needs and putting ourselves first. However, we are taught this is wrong, especially as a parent. But how can you look after a child, if you yourself are running on empty? In a large number of people I have met with post-natal depression, it is because they have been trying to be super-mum-wife-employee-friend-daughter and any other job they are feeling responsible for. They are generally exhausted and feeling very inadequate at every job they are trying to do, often feeling like they are not doing anything well. To try and accomplish every task on their impossible to do lists, they forgo sleep, healthy food, exercise, rest and downtime, all of the essential aspects they need in order to function as a person coping with life. So, if 'being selfish' is a block for you, write yourself a self-care plan for when you become a parent, on how you will fit in your *you* time and be a parent. This is not selfish, it is essential.

'My parents were useless, I will be the same.'

A fear of people from unhappy families is that they will repeat the mistakes of their parents. There is a strong belief that parenting abilities are genetic, but this just simply isn't true. Particularly if you are aware of the issue and take steps to address it prior to becoming a parent. Looking at the situation with empathy and understanding will go a long way towards forgiveness and letting go for you. For example, if your parent worked excessively, perhaps this is why they weren't around a lot. But perhaps they had to do that to provide food and shelter and keep you well cared for. If your parent was not loving or nurturing, perhaps they had closed-off parents that were the same, and they did not know how to nurture and show love to you. Acceptance that they were doing the best they could, but lacked the insight to improve this, will help you. Especially as by reading this, you are showing you do possess that insight to recognise this could be an issue and are taking steps to address i

'My parent was abusive, what if I end up being the same?'

This is a really big fear for people that have come from an abusive family. I have often heard, 'My dad used to hit my mum and me, what if I end up doing the same?' Through healing sessions with these clients, it generally doesn't take long for them to see they are not their parent, that they have a different personality and coping mechanisms to deal with stress. If you are a person that struggles with issues of anger and lashing out, then get professional help to deal with this. Hitting your partner or child is never okay. If you are a person that holds a deep fear you could be this person, then also get help with that. Not only will it prevent you from turning into the abusive person, but it will help you to enjoy your family instead of living in fear of an event that will most probably never happen. Often when trying so hard not to be that angry person, you might find you go too far the other way, and struggle with discipline and healthy boundaries. In my experience, it is the fear that leads to the actual experience, not genetics or anything else.

'I already have one child, I can't possible love another child as much as this one.'

This is often a secret held fear. That all-consuming love you feel for your first child is so intense, that you cannot perceive how you could ever feel that way about another person ever again. But believe me, you can. You will love all of your children just as much as the first, regardless of if you have two or ten. If this is a fear or belief of yours, then definitely use EFT to overcome it. Don't let it stop you from having your second child.

'I wasn't taught how to love or nurture, I won't know how to do it.'

We can learn how to love and nurture, even if we were not shown it as a child. Talk about this with your partner, your in-laws, your friends, anyone you admire for their parenting abilities. Watch them interact with their children, note what you think is good or not something you would want to do. Learn from observing. Do some journaling on the type of parent you want to be. Brain-storm ways you can show love and nurturing that you are comfortable with and incorporate these into your parenting style.

'I don't know anything about kids or being a parent, I can't do it.'

Again, this is something you can learn. No child comes with a how-to-guidebook. Watching people you admire, observing how they do it and also how *not* to do it will go a long way in helping with this belief. Write a list of your values that as a parent you would like to teach your children. Consider the types of discipline you think are appropriate and you are comfortable with. Journal any fears you have of specific things you do not know and then research them. This will teach you a lot about being a parent and remove this particular block, and will have you well prepared for when your baby arrives.

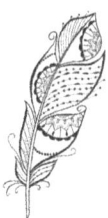

Journaling: drawing out your feelings

Write down all of the things that you are worried about with being a parent. Your list may include items from above, or anything else that comes up for you. If you can, explore ten positive reasons you have for being a parent as well. If you can think of more, I urge you to write more.

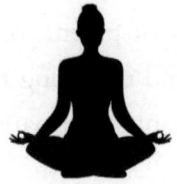

Meditation: for ability to parent

Our ability to be a good parent can be a big fear for many people, particularly if there haven't been good role models in your own life. My belief is we can choose to be the kind of parent we want to be. We can make a conscious decision to follow or not follow those that have come before us. We can take complete responsibility for who we are, and how we parent. This meditation focuses on being a good parent and is suitable for both men and women.

Find a comfortable position for this meditation. You might like to lie down with a pillow under your head and a nice warm blanket. Once you're comfortable, become aware of your breathing. Bring your breathing deeper... breathing deeply... right down past your lungs and into your abdomen. Then slowly and gently, let the breath back out. Notice how the breath fills your lungs completely... right down to your tummy, deep... deep breaths. And notice how gently it turns and slowly leaves, out through your mouth... continue to breathe in this way.

Become aware of a gentle feather brushing the top of your head. Notice that where the feather touches, any stress or tension gets swept away. Feel the feather coming down over the top of your head, and around the back of your head... down over your forehead, your eyebrows, your eyes... your nose, your cheeks, your ears... across your mouth and around your jaw, down to your chin. Feel all the stress start to leave your body with the touch of that feather. Feel the feather go down over your neck… in between your shoulder blades, and down across your shoulders… down your arms, past your elbows down to your wrists and to the tips of your fingers. Feel the feather gently brush down past your chest, down your back and your sides, across your tummy… around your buttock and into your legs. Feel all the tension just be swept away as the feather gently brushes down your legs, past your knees, your calves and into your ankles… down to the tips of your toes. Notice how heavy and relaxed your body feels.

Now see yourself standing in a beautiful park… smell the fresh green grass… feel the sun on your face, a gentle breeze… you hear the happy laughter of a child, and as you look around you recognise your child running towards you… notice how you feel seeing this beautiful being you created coming towards you… notice how you respond… do you lift your child into the air… perhaps you crouch down next to him or her, as they show you something exciting they found in the park… notice how you talk, the tone of your voice, the words you use… notice how easily you connect with your child, how natural it feels to hug and love them…

As you run around and play with your child, you notice they fall over onto the grass and they look to you to see what happens next… notice how you reassure them… provide comfort… show your child they are safe and loved… notice how effortlessly you care for this little being… how easy it is to love them…

You play for a little longer and your child picks up a stick off the ground and throws it at you… they think they are playing but you know it could hurt someone… notice how carefully you respond… how easily you find it to provide discipline in a caring and loving way… notice your child listen and take your words in, a lesson learnt in a way that is empowering and heart felt...

When you are finished playing for the day, you pick your child up and carry them towards home as they chat happily to you about the day and all of the exciting things they saw at the park... all of the fun they had with you... beautiful memories created between you and your child...

As you see yourself bath your child and tuck them into bed that night... notice how you feel... how capable you are of caring for this little human you helped create and bring into the world... spend a few moments enjoying this feeling...

When you are ready, become aware again now of your breathing. Take a few deep breaths, down into your tummy... and gently let them out. Become aware of where your body meets the floor, perhaps at your heels, or the backs of your legs... Your buttock and your back. The backs of your arms or your hands... And the back of your head. Just give your feet and your hands a gently wiggle, as you feel the life reawaken in you. Become aware of any sounds in the room around you... as you gently wake up. When you are ready you can open your eyes, ready to face the day and all the wonderful things it could bring.

CHAPTER SIX
EMOTIONS AS ENERGY

"I take responsibility for my energy and my emotions."

There is a saying 'mind your own energy'. We are not taught a great deal about our body's energy system, and unless we go looking for this information, we may never know it. But we feel it. Have you ever noticed when you are standing next to a person and immediately feel uncomfortable around them? This is your energy mixing with their energy, and it gives you a signal that this person is not good for you. Likewise, when you are around someone who is positive, uplifting, and fun, you feel great, and want to stand closer to them, to bask in their energy.

The energy we put out has a big impact on the energy we get back. Have you heard of that little thing called the Law of Attraction? So, if you are walking around with an energy that is full of blame and resentment, that keeps you being a victim and hard done by, guess what you will get more of? There will always be people with circumstances better or worse than yours. Don't compare your life to anyone else's, you don't know what happens behind closed doors. We only ever see what people choose to show us. The happy person you see out with their new born baby, with their hair and makeup done beautifully, smiling and graceful, might go home and cry for the rest of the day because of the effort it took to go out in the world. The couple with the new baby that look like they have it all made, may be close to bankruptcy for their repeated IVF cycles.

My point is, you never know what anyone else has gone through, or is going through, so be kind. Release your judgements. You no longer need those.

Just as you are affected by the energy of those around you, you affect the energy of everyone you are around. Take responsibility for your energy always and lift it when it needs it. Changing your energy, and changing what you are attracting, will go a long way to changing your situation. This does not mean to 'pretend' to be happy and optimistic all the time. Be real. If you feel hurt, be hurt. If you feel angry, be angry. But don't get stuck there. Feel it, process it, learn from it, then let it go and move on.

People will make mistakes, it is human nature, and it is how we learn and grow. If someone has done something wrong by you, instead of blaming them, look at what was happening in your life at the time. What was your mood and self-talk like? What was the energy you were putting out in to the world at that time? Where do you need to take responsibility, what do you need to learn, and what can you let go? Holding on to anger, resentment and blame will eventually present in your physical body as pain or illness, so it is vital you process these emotions and let them go.

You might find yourself blaming someone else for your circumstances, even though they may not be able to help the situation. I see this a lot for the women who have partners with little or no sperm. It is understandable that you may feel anger or resentment when you can't achieve what you so desperately want because of something they can't provide. But if you can change your perspective, and look at it from the angle of you chose this person to share this journey with you, so what is the lesson here for you, where is the opportunity for self-growth, where can you take responsibility in this situation, then you not only lose that victim energy, but your relationship will be better for it as well.

An easy way of lifting your vibration and changing your life is gratitude. Find gratitude for all of the good things in your life, no matter how small or seemingly insignificant. Be grateful that you wake up in the morning, that you have a house to live in, a job to support you, food to eat. Be grateful for the car park near the shopping centre, the dollar you found on the pavement, the kind word spoken by a stranger. There are so many things to be grateful for in everyday life, but sometimes we have to remind ourselves to look.

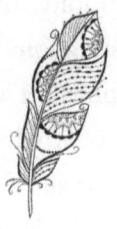

Journaling: changing your vibration

Are there other areas of your life that you can identify where you see yourself as a victim or hard done by? You don't need to judge yourself here, simply become aware, take the steps to process these feelings, so you can change your vibration.

1. Identify the areas and write about these.
2. Create a gratitude list. Make this a daily ritual.

Become aware every day of when you complain or judge. Simply acknowledge these thoughts and stop them in their tracks. Have an affirmation you can use at these times such as:

"I forgive myself for this thought, I'm choosing to let it go and view this person/situation from a place of love instead."

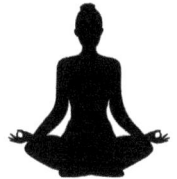

Meditation: for support

A lack of support can be a big fear for a lot of women during pregnancy and motherhood. This could be a result of being a single mum, perhaps your own mother is not around or not supportive. You may have a partner and yet still feel unsupported. It might be from not having friends that have children yet, or any other number of reasons. There is a saying it takes a village to raise a child, and this is true to a degree. Feeling unsupported for long periods of time can take its toll physically and emotionally. This meditation focuses on identifying the support you do have and creating a feeling of support by connecting to your own inner strength and divine source, or whatever it is you hold faith in.

Lie comfortably with your head rested on a pillow, use a blanket if you need too, to keep warm. Become aware of your breathing and observe how it starts to slow down as you begin to relax. Start to deepen your in-breaths, deep down into your abdomen, and just as slowly... release the breath as you exhale. Concentrate on your breathing for a few moments, slowly in... and slowly out... Feel any tension starting to leave your body. Starting at the tip of your head... relax your face and down your neck. Relax your chest and your back... slowly down your arms. Let the relaxation travel down your spine... your tummy, your back. Feel your hips relax... your buttocks. Relax down through the tops of your legs, over your knees, your lower legs and your feet… to the tip of your toes. Notice how relaxed your whole body feels, heavy against the floor or chair.

In your mind's eye, see yourself standing in a field. It's a beautiful field… you can smell the fresh flowers… feel the green grass soft under your feet… the sun is shining in the blue sky and you feel the warmth on your skin… there is a refreshing cool breeze that gently lifts your hair… you raise your face to the sky…. Eyes closed… Holding your arms out… notice how safe you feel here… how free… spend a few moments here simply enjoying the silence… your own company… feeling completely supported by all of the elements of nature… standing tall and strong… open to possibility… allow joy to fill you… peace… know there is nowhere else you need to be right now…

When you are ready you open your eyes… you sense someone standing near you… they are safe… supportive… as you turn to face them, simply notice who they are. This might be someone in your life now, someone who was previously in your life… or maybe they symbolise the person you would like in your life… they ask you now what you need? Take your time in replying… let any answer that comes to mind flow from your lips free of judgement… it's okay to want help… it's okay to want to feel supported… take your time and tell them everything you need in your life…

When you have finished, let your mind wander to the people who are in your life… those who do support you. It might be a partner… a parent… a friend… a colleague… they might support you in big ways or small… as you think of each person that supports you in some way, see them join you in the field… try not to force this… just allow the ideas and thoughts to come… if you are having trouble thinking of people, try to imagine the type of person you would like in your life and how they would support you… it might be the supermarket worker that offers to carry your bags to the car… it might be a supportive neighbour that brings your bins in… as you think of more and more people that could support you in life, bring them into the field with you… take as long as you need here…

When you are ready, look around the field and see all of the faces of all of the people ready to support you… see them smiling at you, and smile back… send gratitude and love to every single person that supports you in any way, not matter how big or small…

As you thank each of these people they leave the field until you are standing there alone once more, but feeling loved and supported… you might like to sit down now in the field, and as you close your eyes gently, you become aware of a different kind of being nearby… a supportive being that is a direct connection to universal source… it might be a loved one who has passed, your higher self, an angel, God… any divine source you feel a connection to… as they take a seat in front of you they look you deep in the eyes and ask you what you need… again take your time replying… how can this divine source assist you… perhaps they can send you signs to guide you throughout the day… perhaps they can send you helpful people… maybe it's just an angelic hug in the times that are hard… spend as much time as you need now talking to this angelic being, this divine source…

When you feel ready, you thank the being for coming here to support you today and know they will be with you always… know that in the future you can take a few quiet moments to connect with this Divine source whenever you are needing help or guidance…as you prepare to leave the field, take a moment to acknowledge any guidance or messages you have received here today..

Notice your breathing now… Become aware of the sounds in the room around you. Gently wriggle your fingers and toes… Take a nice deep breath in and as you exhale, open your eyes.

CHAPTER SEVEN
EMOTIONAL AWARENESS

"It is safe to examine my emotions."

Is there a reason you don't want to get pregnant?

This sounds like a very silly question, when assumedly you are reading this book because you want to have a baby. But we do often have underlying fears, beliefs, or emotions that stop us from getting pregnant. We have explored this in detail throughout the book, but before we move on, let's look at some very basic concepts.

If I told you, hypothetically, that you would definitely get pregnant if you:

- Cut out all processed foods.
- Lost weight.
- Chart your mucous daily.
- Practice daily self-care measures such as meditation, yoga and tapping exercises.
- Walked around the block every single day.
- Stopped smoking/drinking/any other unhealthy lifestyle choice.
- Stopped blaming anyone else and took complete responsibility for everything in your life.

… would you do it?

If you said no to any of these things, then you need to ask yourself why not? If the thing you want most in the world is to have a baby, why would you not take every possible healthy step to achieve it?

There are a lot of perceived downsides to having a baby as well. Here is a list of just a few that I have come across, but I'm sure there are many more.

- I will get fat.
- I don't want stretch marks.
- I will lose my freedom.
- I won't be able to travel.
- I will need time off work, I can't afford that.
- It will hurt (labour).
- It could go wrong, and that would be too painful.
- My partner isn't kind, I don't want that for my child.

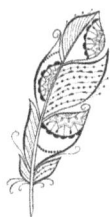

Journaling: feelings for pregnancy

1. Did you say no to any of the questions? If so, write these down and explore the reasons you don't want to do them; you might be surprised by the answers.

2. If you said yes to all of them, are you doing them already? If not, write down why you are not doing them, or if you really believe this is an honest answer, start doing these things every single day. If you don't, you have a block here and you need to explore that.

3. Did any of the downsides of having a baby resonate with you? Do you have others? Write about this and be very honest with yourself. No-one else needs to read this, but it is important you process these feelings and beliefs.

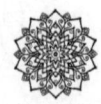

CHAPTER EIGHT
FINDING HAPPINESS BEFORE THE BABY

"My happiness is my responsibility."

Many people think they will be happy once they have a baby. I did. We assume we are only unhappy because we are infertile. That having a baby will fix everything, and we will be happy, and our lives will be perfect. While for some people, there may be some truth in this, however for the vast majority having a baby may not bring the happiness you thought it would. Once the baby arrives, it's hard work, you're tired, there could be financial constraints, there can be arguments over family roles, or if you're single you might resent never getting a break.

It's important to find happiness before the baby.

When trying to conceive, it can very quickly become the full focus of your life. Every second of every day is spent thinking about getting pregnant. Changing plans or not making plans because you might be pregnant is common. Continuous Google searches on infertility and how best to deal with it become all-consuming. Harassing your partner for sex even when he does not want to perform creates anger, resentment and a very big breakdown in a relationship.

It is always an idea to educate yourself and make appropriate changes to your health and life style in order to prepare for a pregnancy and parenthood. However, if your behaviour becomes obsessive this needs to be addressed. When we *need* something in an obsessive way, we create the opposite effect of repelling it.

I have seen people take a break from IVF treatments, or 'honestly give up' on becoming pregnant, only to find they are pregnant the following cycle naturally. I say 'honestly give up' here, because pretending you have given up just to trick the Universe into getting you pregnant doesn't work.

When planning a pregnancy, women often put their lives on hold just in case they are pregnant or have a new born. This could be as simple as not booking concert tickets, or not planning that trip of a lifetime. It could be bigger life changes such as turning down a job promotion or not buying that house or car. Putting your life on hold will not create the happy, fulfilled life you are seeking. If you end up having a baby, you will make it work. Accepting the job promotion doesn't mean you have to stay in that job, you can always change again if it doesn't work around having a baby. You can postpone the holiday you booked but can't take because you have a newborn. It is vital to keep living your life. Assume that a baby, or a few, will be a part of your life, but don't stop living in anticipation of that day. Live your life as though it is inevitable, and you can do it all. If it turns out you can't, you can make the necessary changes when you need to.

I believe a major block to happiness is stress. We will discuss this in detail in chapter nine, but there are some aspects of stress to start considering before we move forward. We often live in a constant state of stress. This increases cortisone in our body and creates a fight or flight response. The fight or flight response is our bodies way of protecting us when confronted with danger. Unfortunately, we often stay in this response and it doesn't get switched off like it should. When we are faced with danger, the body systems that are not required in that moment of stress to keep us alive are turned off. This includes our digestive system—we will not be eating when running away from a bear for example—and, also our reproductive system as we will not be having sex and creating babies whilst running away from a bear. Staying in this heightened state of stress nevertheless, keeps these systems switched off.

Often women don't identify stress in their lives or their bodies well. However, if you are tracking your cycle, you might see the fertile mucous appear and then disappear without ovulation occurring, or your oestrogen levels may increase only to decrease again, creating long cycles or infertile cycles. This is very often a response to stress in your body. You may have had a difficult day at the office, you may have not eaten properly for a few days, the body sees starvation as a response to a threat because you have been too busy or are trying to lose weight, you may have started a new rigorous exercise program, and while the intention is correct, over doing it is just as unhelpful. You may have had an argument with a friend, or money concerns. There are so many possible causes in everyday life for stress, and yet we often 'power on' and don't identify this.

A very simple technique for resetting the flight or fight response is focusing on your breath as you slow your breathing. Breathing in slowly, breathing out slowly. We don't realise how often we hold our breath or take shallow or rapid breathes because we are so focused on our to-do list, or unconsciously responding to our environment or emotions. If you forget to do this breathing exercise regularly, set your alarm for every hour on the hour, and count to 5 as you breathe in, count to 5 as you breathe out, and do this cycle of breathwork 5 times. Or commit to doing it every time you go to the toilet, or any other activity you do several times a day. Do it when you wake up and before you go to sleep, do it in the shower. Just make conscious breathing a habit.

If you need more help in creating more positivity and passion in your life, you might like to purchase my book, *Using Positivity to Make a Better Life* available on Amazon. It contains several simple, but effective techniques to make healthy changes in your life.

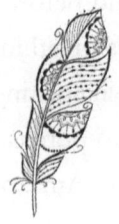

Journaling: identifying feelings for happiness

1. Identify ways you are obsessing about pregnancy or fertility and write these down.
2. Identify areas or causes of stress in your life.
3. If you track your cycles, notice where they indicate a stress response.
4. Have you put any areas of your life on hold anticipating a pregnancy or a baby?

Once you have done this, I want you to try something that might be very difficult and will likely take practice and perseverance. I want you to set your intention of a pregnancy, don't limit it to dates and times, write this down, and then let it go, and simply trust it will happen.

Then, find a new focus for your life that creates passion and excitement for you. It most likely will be something creative: singing, dancing, knitting, classes on something new like cooking, or learning a language. You want an outlet for your stress that you enjoy and look forward to. That makes you smile when you think about doing it. You might want to book a holiday, or go for that job promotion, or enrol in a course.

If you can include your partner in this passion even better, it will help take both your minds off the fertility issue, unite you together in fun and strengthen your relationship. This might be kayaking down a river or taking dance classes together. It might be setting a 'date day' every week or month, where you go out to the movies and to dinner. Romance will flow more easily and allow sex to be fun again and not a chore that divides you.

This will raise your energetic vibrations and take the responsibility off pregnancy for being your only source of happiness and create new avenues for happiness and igniting passion in your life. Often times, pregnancy is a happy side-effect!

Write a list of things that make you happy. How often do you do these things? Can you start doing them more?

CHAPTER NINE
RELEASING STRESS AND GUILT

"I remind myself to breathe..."

Stress is a very important topic. Women generally are not great at identifying when they're stressed either, which doesn't help in making changes that are needed.

When talking about stress it's vital to understand the fight or flight response. This is a response to danger, real or perceived, that kicks in when we recognise a stress or danger, so we can fight or get away. This process is supposed to keep us safe and alive. Once the stress or danger has passed the flight or fight response should switch off and our body should return to normal function. However, in this modern age this doesn't always happen. We function at a constant level of stress and the response never turns off. We get through our days in a constant state of fight or flight.

This can have short- and long-term effects on our health. The fight or flight response results in an influx of adrenaline and cortisol in our bodies. Our non-vital body systems get turned off as we discussed in chapter eight. Increased adrenaline levels cause our heart to race, our blood pressure goes up and our breathing changes. Our blood gets shunted from organs to muscles, preparing us to run. Increased cortisol affects our weight and our reproductive system amongst other things. Your eye sight changes, your vision narrows, and your hearing becomes more sensitive. Your body is on alert ready to fight or run away. This is a great response if you are actually in danger, but what if you're not? What if you think you are, and your body thinks you are, but actually you're not?

Think about that state of panic and fear for a moment. Now imagine functioning at that level for most of your day. Think of your typical day. Your morning might consist of being woken by an alarm clock before your body is ready to wake up. You might realise you forgot to iron a uniform the day before, or perhaps you've run out of milk and bread. You might get an unexpected phone call that makes you run late. You might be thinking ahead of what you have to do for the day, worrying you will be late for work, fearing reprimands from your boss, you might have to get through traffic, there could be a lot of it, making you later. Perhaps a car swerves in front of you and you have to slam your foot on the break! You finally get to work, you may or may not get in trouble from your boss but either way the fear remains. Perhaps you have a stressful day, dealing with angry or impatient clients or colleagues, you get a five-minute break where you scoff your lunch instead of having an actual break. Your digestive system has switched off, so the food sits in your stomach making you feel sick and lethargic. The work day finally finishes, and you are already thinking ahead about preparing a meal, maybe you need to go to the shop first and what are you going to cook? It could be a battle between nutrition, cost and just simply getting something on the table. After tea you have to do the dishes, you remember there is no clean uniform for the next day, so you need to wash, dry and iron before you can go to bed. You remember you had to do some reading for work the next day, the bins need to go out and you forgot to ring the mechanic again about that noise your car is making. Perhaps hubby wants some special attention before you go to sleep (a vital component if you're trying to have a baby)! You do a quick tidy up of the house noting the rest will have to wait until the weekend. You make a mental note of everything you need to do the following day, you go to bed, you have a restless sleep because your mind can't switch off. You get up the next morning to the sounds of the alarm, and you start all over again.

The stress response may have turned off briefly while you slept, but it most probably didn't return to baseline, and it was probably straight back up in the morning. Your body is constantly stressed, your adrenaline and cortisol remain elevated, you're constantly on the lookout for perceived or potential dangers. Your body is set to fight ... every minute of the day. This amazing mechanism your body has to keep you alive is slowly killing you, leaving you wide open to illness and a struggling to function body. How long do you think that can continue?

So, what can you do about it? The simplest tool is to breathe! Remind yourself to breathe, slowly, deeply, regularly throughout the day. Find tools that can help, such as meditation, tapping and essential oils. While you are managing your stress levels, you might also need to manage the stress side effects. This could be anything from headaches, poor digestion, irregular menstrual cycles or a lowered immune system.

Using breathing techniques and tapping throughout the day can lower your stress levels. There isn't an overnight fix to turning off the flight or fight response to chronic stress, so you will need to put in a conscious effort initially, until these practices become habits. But you can do it, and it is worth it.

Recognising your stress and naming it is important. It's vital to know that you are stressed, but do you really figure out why, or is it just a pile of different things that add up and become overwhelming? Identifying what your stressors are and naming them can be really helpful. Ask yourself, why am I feeling so stressed? It might be that a car cut you off on your way to work and you're angry, thinking about what could have happened. You relive it all day long, ruminate over it which may create stress in other areas of your life. Acknowledging your anger as soon as it happens, reminding yourself to breathe, reassure yourself that while it could have been worse, thankfully it was not, then let it go and move on with your day.

Tracking your cycle is a great way to also monitor your stress. If you find ovulation is getting postponed, your cycles are becoming irregular or non-existent check in with your stress levels.

Your body will let you know when it's stressed. Recognising and observing the signs is really important for your cycles and your overall health. Stress could appear in your body in many different ways. A change in sleep patterns is a common one. Difficulty falling asleep, waking overnight, waking too early and still feeling tired, or struggling to wake up when you need to are all signs of stress. Upsetting or restless dreams can be a sign your mind is trying to process things from your day that you are not recognising or dealing with. If you sleep all night but wake feeling exhausted, it's likely you are having a restless sleep even if you don't remember your dreams.

Pain in the body can be another sign of stress. Aching or sore muscles and joints, headaches or neck stiffness, or generally feeling like you are many years older than you actually are can all be signs of chronic stress. If you find yourself becoming prone to injuries and illness check in with your stress levels.

Mood swings and lack of focus or concentration are all signs of acute or chronic stress. If you struggle to find the right words, use the incorrect words or forget what you're saying mid-sentence it could be simply tiredness or exhaustion secondary to stress. If you forget to do things or find yourself walking into a room in your house but no idea why you're there, that can be stress. If you are moody, irritable, lacking patience, developing a short temper or lacking motivation to do things that are good for you it's probably because you are stressed.

If your digestion and bowel habits are changing this can be a sign of acute or chronic stress too. Constipation or diarrhoea, nausea, reflux, bloating and craving unhealthy foods can all be contributed to stress.

Please be mindful that all of these could also be indicative of other health issues, so if any of these signs and symptoms are presenting in your life, please have them checked out by a medical professional.

Sometimes the ways in which we 'manage' our stress also do more harm than good. For example, you might need several coffees to get through the day and a glass of wine (or several) to wind down at the end of the day. Perhaps you smoke in order to have breaks throughout the day, or your vice might be chocolate bars. You might become dependent on prescription medications to manage the pain or to try and sleep. This isn't to say you can't ever have a coffee or a wine or chocolate bar, but when you *need* them to function this is a problem. Most of these 'tools' for managing your stress can create further stress and side effects and exacerbate the problems you are trying to address.

I had a patient who had terrible cycles. They were irregular, and her oestrogen levels didn't get very high. She tried for a pregnancy for several months and nothing was happening. She was angry and sad. She took a month off and when she returned, she looked different. Her face was brighter, she was calmer, and her cycle had improved. When I asked her what had changed, she said she had been looking into the effects of stress on fertility and had joined a meditation group. The change in her was incredible and she went on to become pregnant effortlessly.

Guilt also affects us in many different ways. I quite often see clients who are suffering guilt from a wide range of causes and unfortunately this affects their health in many ways. Fertility is often one of them depending on the cause of the guilt.

People experience guilt for an array of reasons. It can be from something they have done, thought or wished for. It can be from something that has been done to them by another person. It can even be for something you didn't realise you had done, but someone else has made sure you feel and own the guilt you are 'responsible' for. Or it could be a third-party putting guilt on you for something you didn't even do. Human emotions are complicated, and people are complicated. Not everything is based on logic or fact.

Guilt affecting fertility can be from having sex at a young age, where it was not permitted by your parents, church, or other authority figures. This can lead to the person believing they are 'bad' or 'undeserving' of good things in life. Sex later in life outside of your marriage, or perhaps with someone else who is married or committed to another person, can also lead to these same feelings of unworthiness.

Guilt can likewise be the result of what someone else has done to you, and sadly this is often abuse of some sort. We will explore this in more detail later. Unfortunately, the victim in abuse is often the one left feeling the guilt for the abuse. People who never talk about it, or never have the abuse validated by the perpetrator or an authority figure (such as their parents or the legal system) tend to experience the guilt even more profusely. They often think they 'deserved' it or 'asked for it'. Sometimes they feel like they were the *other* woman despite never consenting to the abuse. These all lead to the same feelings of being a bad and undeserving person, and no bad or undeserving person is entitled to something as great as being a parent, are they?

Sometimes you may not feel guilty for something you have done, because you have worked through it in your own mind and dealt with it, or perhaps you know the 'full story' where others do not. However, if a third-party finds out, they can often take the moral high ground and attempt to make sure you feel the guilt, and this can lead you questioning yourself and your actions, despite the healing work you have already put in. This brings a whole other level of complication to your situation, and while you don't have your own guilt affecting your fertility, the beliefs and opinions of others affects it instead. 'They said I don't deserve to be happy because of what I did ... maybe they are right.'

It might be that another person involved won't let you forget what you did and move on. For their story to continue they need your guilt to continue. At some point though, you both need to let it go and move on, either together or separately, for your own health and wellbeing.

Now, let's look at guilt from a different perspective. What if it was your partner that cheated on you? Do you continue to blame them and make them pay for their mistake? In this way not getting pregnant works as a punishment for their behaviour. In this instance I would highly recommend getting marriage counselling. You don't want to bring a baby into this scenario until you have resolved it.

Guilt can also come about if you are the person in the relationship that has a health issue affecting your fertility. If the male has a poor sperm count for example, or if the female has PCOS or endometriosis. There can be a lot of guilt and this is something you will likely need to work through together.

Sometimes you simply need to forgive yourself or others. Learning from mistakes is important and not repeating those mistakes is also very important. However, most people will make a mistake of some kind in their life, often many. That doesn't mean you have to 'pay' for them forever. If you make the decision to stay in the relationship you need to find a way to move on and not hold onto the guilt or the blame.

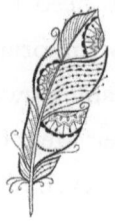

Journal: writing out stressors and guilt

1. What causes stress in your life?

2. How do you currently manage stress? Is it effective? Healthy or unhealthy?

3. In what ways does your body show you that you're stressed?

4. What are some new ways you can start to manage your stress more effectively?

5. Write a plan to check in daily with your stress (recognition is vital), and any unhealthy 'tools' you are reliant on. Now consider new ways to manage your stress level. Commit to at least three things. Come back to this list as you read through the book and learn new techniques.

6. Are there times in your life when you have done something you are not proud of? Are they your opinions or do they belong to someone else? What have you done to learn and grow from these mistakes?

7. Can you see how these experiences are still affecting your life today? Explore this and write them all down.

8. Now go through the list, and for every point you have written, forgive yourself or the other person involved.

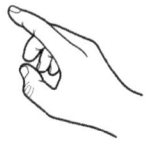

Tapping Script 3: for stress

This is a very quick tapping you can use if you are stressing out and feeling overwhelmed and need to calm yourself down quickly.

The karate chop point (KP): Even though I am feeling very stressed,

I love and accept myself deeply and completely.

The karate point: Even though I feel overwhelmed at what I need to achieve today,

I am okay.

The karate point: Even though I can feel my heart racing and it's difficult to breathe,

I am supported, I have the tools in place to cope, I am okay.

Inner Eye (IE): I am stressed

Outer Eye (OE): am stressing out

Under Eye (UE): This is too much

Under Nose (UN): It's all too hard

Under Mouth (UM): I can't keep going

Collarbone (CB) *use fist*: I want to quit

Under Arm (UA) *use hand*: I can't do it all by myself

Top of the Head (TH): I'm feeling completely overwhelmed

Inner Eye (IE): I am okay

Outer Eye (OE): Breathe

Under Eye (UE): I am calming my body down

Under Nose (UN): My body is just trying to keep me safe and that's why my heart is racing. Include and any other physical symptoms.

Under Mouth (UM): I am safe

Collarbone (CB): Breathe ... *slow your breathing*

Under Arm (UA): I am okay

Top of the Head (TH): I'm breathing ... *slower still*

CHAPTER TEN
RELATIONSHIPS FOR FERTILITY

"I am worthy of a healthy and loving relationship."

If you are in a relationship, it is worth looking at how healthy it is.

If you are in a loving and respectful relationship, is there anything that is *not* quite right? Are there any areas of your relationship that hold doubt for either of you? If so, take the time to explore this and try to overcome it. Sometimes simply having a good and honest conversation is enough. Sometimes you may need to seek the assistance of a professional third party.

If your relationship is unhealthy or unhappy, bringing a child into the mix will not fix it. More than likely, it will add to the stress and the strain that is already present. I have had many people say to me that they are so desperate for a child, that they do not have the time to leave a relationship and hopefully find another one that will in more time result in having a child. It sometimes seems like a better option to stay in an unhappy relationship in order to have a child. If you are fighting and unhappy, is that the environment that a baby wants to be in? Is this the person that you can discuss your ideas on parenting, schooling, health and every other aspect of a child's life, for the rest of your life? Is this the relationship you want to model to your children for them to aspire to when they are older? If not, can your relationship be improved? If both parties want to save the relationship, then hopefully with love, kindness, respect and perhaps professional help, the relationship can be improved and made happy once more. If not, then a better choice would perhaps be to leave the unhealthy relationship, focusing on your wants and needs, and attracting a relationship that is more suitable to those. Choosing to stay in order to have children may prove to be very difficult later in life if you decide to separate and have to share custody of your children. If your marriage is already on the rocks, considering all future possibilities now may save you a lot of grief in the future.

It is never a good idea to bring a child into an abusive relationship, and if this is the situation you have found yourself in, please seek professional assistance to remove yourself from the relationship. Unfortunately, domestic violence is very common, and sometimes it builds over time, and therefore you don't even realise it has begun, let alone how it happened. I can *not* stress enough, to please get help, if this is your situation.

If you are single, does this cause you concern for raising a child? I know some single women that are more than happy to be a single parent. I know others that are saddened at not having another person to share the joys and hardships of parenting with. Either situation is okay, so long as you are okay with it.

While researching for this book, I had a client we will refer to simply as K. K was in a very unhappy marriage with an alcoholic. She experienced several pregnancies, and equal number of miscarriages throughout her marriage. She looks back now and realises that her body was protecting her from bringing a child into this very unstable environment, and from being attached to this man for the rest of her life. Fortunately for K, she was eventually able to leave the marriage, and had a successful pregnancy resulting in twins with a new and loving partner.

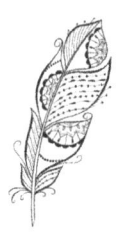

Journaling: for fertile grounds

Are you currently in a relationship? If so, do you consider it a healthy relationship? Spend some time now doing some automatic writing about your relationship. Explore what is good, and what is perhaps not so good. Use these questions to help you journal your feelings.

1. Do you share the same ideas and beliefs around raising children?
2. Do you agree on vaccinations, circumcision, discipline, schooling, religion?
3. Do you want children equally?
4. Do you harbour any doubts about your relationship or your ability to raise children successfully within it?

If your writing brings up any areas of concern, try talking to your partner about these, see if you can resolve them together. Consider seeking professional help in the form of a counsellor if you need more help.

If you are single, this is a good time to look at the type of relationship you do want, if you want one.

1. What will it look like?
2. How will you treat each other?
3. What aspects are important to you in a relationship?
4. Will your new partner accept a child you have conceived via IVF?
5. What role would a new partner play in the parenting of your child?

CHAPTER ELEVEN
SINGLE WOMEN AND SAME-SEX COUPLES

"Being a mother is my birthright."

Being a single parent no longer has the stigma associated it with it that it once did. Women can be proactive now and choose to start a family's when they're ready. There's no more waiting around for Mr Right, or settling for Mr Right now. Single women or same-sex couples have an obvious fertility issue—a lack of sperm—which can be easily resolved using a sperm donor. Nevertheless, often these ladies don't have successful pregnancies straight away, and this causes them a lot of distress and loss of hope. The assumption generally is that pregnancy should happen easily, as they don't have fertility issues other than not having a male counterpart to create a baby. Their cycles are monitored closely, the sperm or embryo is inserted at exactly the right time of the month. Therefore, it is a valid assumption that pregnancy should occur.

For single and same-sex coupled women, I have found there are a variety of emotional issues that affect their pregnancy success rates. In addition to the causes already discussed throughout this book, these women face a multitude of other issues. All of these issues are based in the woman's belief system. These may well be her own beliefs, or they may be inherited beliefs from their parents or grandparents, or perhaps simply a fear of what the beliefs of anyone around them will be.

These are some of the most common beliefs I have witnessed, but I'm sure there are many others:

Use of donor sperm

Not knowing the donor – a child should know his/her father.

What will you tell the child as he/she grows up about his/her father?

What will people think? A one-night stand, promiscuity?

Raising a child alone

It has been a long-accepted belief of general society that it takes two to create a baby. And if you do not have a partner, then the option of parenthood is closed to you. However, with today's technology it is really quite simple and affordable to achieve a pregnancy without a partner. Nonetheless, going down this road raises all sorts of questions and concerns. For example, a woman considering being a single mum might ask herself,

- Do I really want to do this on my own? To not have someone else to share the joys, the concerns, the night feeds, the responsibility?
- Am I capable of doing it on my own?
- What will people think if I don't have a partner? Will they assume I am promiscuous?
- What if I finally meet someone and they're not interested because I have a child?
- Can I afford this on my own?
- How can I work and be a mum?

Addressing any of these issues is a vital step in considering becoming a single mum, because nature has a way of protecting us, so doubt could have an effect on your pregnancy success if you are unsure if this is the correct path for you to take.

Beliefs about a same-sex person having a child

A woman in a lesbian relationship faces the above issues regarding donor sperm, as well as others. Ladies in a same-sex relationship have discussed the following areas of concern with me, but again I am sure there are plenty more beliefs and judgements out there.

- I gave up the right to be a parent when I 'chose' to be a lesbian.
- Children deserve a mother and a father.
- If I have children, they also will be gay.
- My children will be teased at school for having *two* mums.
- The idea of using a man's sperm is too uncomfortable for me to consider.

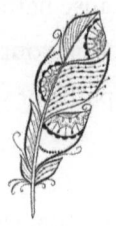

Journaling: for clarity on your fertility path

Consider all of the questions, beliefs or judgements raised in this chapter. Which ones apply to you? Are there others that haven't been written here?

Write about these, explore the beliefs and where they come from? Are they yours or some-one else's? Are they factual or a fear that may not eventuate?

CHAPTER TWELVE
IVF, DONORS AND SURROGACY

"I am grateful for all of the options available to me."

If you have a physical condition or illness that prevents you from being able to become pregnant or carry a child, you most likely will consider IVF, and this may also include surrogacy, donor sperm, donor eggs or embryos.

I have a huge respect for science and the possibilities IVF has opened up for people with infertility and the role it plays for single or same-sex couples who cannot conceive on their own. If you need to go down the route of Assisted Reproductive Technology (ART) then do so, but before you spend thousands of dollars, please do everything possible to help your fertility before-hand. Do the exercises in this book, eat well, exercise, lose or gain weight if you need to, have great self-care practices in place and manage your stress. If you get pregnant on your own with some healthy changes, that is fantastic, and if you don't at least you know you are doing everything you possibly can to make your IVF cycle a success.

My apprehension around IVF and ART is in some cases it is becoming more of a business, and less about the person. I am very concerned that using your superannuation is now an option for paying for IVF. Because the success rate of IVF is approximately 8-40%, dependent on many factors such as weight, age, and health conditions, there is a strong possibility that you will not have a child at the end of your IVF journey, and you will also not have any money to retire with. This means large mortgages, working long beyond the age where you wanted to retire, and a whole lot of emotional and financial strain.

While it is a gift to have these options available, it may also create further emotional issues that you will need to recognise and process. This may not apply to everyone going down this path, but they are worth considering. It is a very good idea to set yourself a limit before you start. It may be a time frame, or a specific number of cycles. Once you start it can be very difficult to stop, because statistically the more cycles you do the more likely it is you will achieve a pregnancy. No one wants to stop when the next one could be 'the one'. When people ask me when they should stop, my answer is always the same, 'when you can no longer do it emotionally, physically or financially.'

If you had always assumed your baby would be created by you and your partner, it may be difficult to accept using another woman's eggs or another man's sperm. Issues that may arise are the feeling or belief that this child won't technically be yours, a fear that you may not connect with the child or that it may create a division between you and your partner. These are all valid fears or concerns, and it is really important to acknowledge them if they apply to you. Allow yourself to grieve the loss or hurt, or any other emotion you feel. You can be grateful for what you are receiving while still feeling the loss of how you thought it would be.

Using a surrogate may also bring up these issues and more. There may be the fears mentioned above of feeling like the child isn't yours, or not connecting with the child. You may also have a lot of fear or questions around the role this third person will have in your child's life.

While dealing with the emotional aspects that come up for you, it is also important to have legal advice from someone knowledgeable in this area, so that all parties involved know exactly where they stand *and* understand their rights and responsibilities. This in itself will go a long way towards addressing your fears and concerns.

Depending on the reason for using a surrogate or donor, this may in itself create other beliefs or emotional issues. For example, if you are using a donor because your own eggs are of poor quality, this could create resentment or anger towards your body. Or, if your partner has poor sperm, this could create feelings of anger or resentment towards your partner. Perhaps you had or have a medical condition that makes it necessary, which could possibly create feelings of anger, loss, hurt or feeling hard done by. There could be any number of issues here, so consider them now without any judgement towards yourself or others. Whatever you feel is okay.

What if you have had a medical illness that has caused your infertility? Or perhaps the treatment for the illness has caused your infertility. This is often the case for people that have had illnesses such as cancer.

In this instance, it is worth looking at the emotional causes of the original illness. For example, if you had cervical cancer that required a biopsy, this could make carrying a child difficult, and could result in miscarriages that fall under the broad infertility banner.

According to Inna Segal, cervical cancer presents when the person is feeling out of flow with life, resisting femininity or feeling disrespected as a woman, feeling unwanted, lacking affection or sexual conflict. The woman may feel frustrated because of a lack of commitment or attention in a relationship, feeling ignored, unimportant, useless empty or cheated.

Breast cancer can also often be a reason for needing to use a surrogate, due to the risks of the cancer returning with the increased levels of oestrogen in pregnancy. In Inna Segal's words, she suggests, 'breast cancer is related to the inability to nurture yourself, taking on everyone's problems, feeling guilty or wronged, too much worry and apprehension, a lack of self-confidence and love, or feeling like a victim.'

If you have had another medical issue that has affected your fertility, I would highly recommend Inna Segal's book, *The Secret Language of Your Body* to explore potential emotional causes and use the tools she provides to resolve them. By addressing these issues, you may in fact assist your fertility as well.

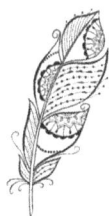

Journaling: for acceptance; thoughts, beliefs

1. If you are considering IVF, write about how you are feeling about this. Remember, it is likely you will have very mixed feelings, so it's important to acknowledge the 'good and bad'. While you might feel grateful for the opportunity, you may feel anger and resentment at needing to do it, you may feel fear around the financial pressures, or any other number of emotions. Explore this in depth to process your emotions.

2. If you are using a surrogate or donor, journal your thoughts, beliefs and feelings around this. Consider the reasons for needing to use a surrogate or donor. What feelings does this bring up for you?

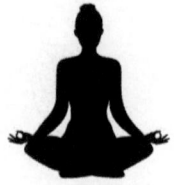

Meditation: for IVF

IVF is a process where eggs are removed directly from the ovaries and fertilised with sperm outside of the body to create embryos, and if they survive, transferred approximately a week later into the woman's uterus, or frozen if they are not being used straight away. Eggs can also be frozen without the use of sperm, which is becoming a common practice for women who are single and getting older but haven't yet met the person they want to have children with. This process is often used when there is a cancer diagnosis and treatment will likely cause the woman to become infertile. In this instance, often the woman will also need to find a surrogate to carry their future children, as pregnancy can be a significant risk factor for oestrogen dominant cancers returning. This meditation focuses on the first stage of IVF, where eggs are removed from the body, and is suitable for women going through IVF. This meditation uses a much shorter relaxation stage, so if you need longer to relax into the meditation, simply replace this section with a relaxation stage from another meditation.

Find yourself a comfortable place to sit or lie down, where you are warm, and your back is supported. Maybe sitting in a chair, or lying on the floor, with a pillow and a blanket. Once you are comfortable, close your eyes and take a nice deep breath in, filling up your lungs with fresh oxygen, all the way down to your tummy. And as you slowly release the breath, feel any tension leaving with it as your body relaxes into the chair or floor beneath you. Again, take another deep breath in, and as the breath turns to leave, feel it picking up your tensions and taking them from your body. Continue to breathe like this for a few moments, breathing in peace and relaxation and breathing out any tension or stress.

Now become aware of a beautiful rainbow light dancing around the top of your head. Swirling around. As it brushes past your skin it picks up and remaining tension dissolving it... and you feel it leave your body. Feel the beautiful vibrant colours of the rainbow, swirl around your head, down over your forehead... across your eyes, your nose, your ears, your cheeks, your mouth and down your jaw. Feel it swirl around your neck and around your shoulders, down both your arms, swirling round your wrists, and your hands and each of your fingers. Feel the rainbow swirling down your trunk... your back, your chest and your sides. Around your buttock and each of your legs, slowly swirling down around past your knees, your calves, your ankles, your feet and each of your toes... As the tension leaves your body feel yourself relaxing heavily into the seat or floor, and the rainbow light just sits softly around you. Relaxing you, keeping you safe and warm, as you continue along this journey.

In your mind's eye bring your attention to your ovaries... see them full of healthy growing follicles... send calm and loving energy to both ovaries now... watch the follicles grow steadily... see an egg within each follicle... Developing as it should... healthy and ready for life... take as much time as you need here... Filling both ovaries with love... you might like to talk to your ovaries... thank them for the amazing job they are doing... for working extra hard this month... you might like to talk to the eggs that are growing... tell them how much they are wanted... how much you love them and are grateful to them for simply being... (You might want to do this stage several times during the start of your treatment before going to theatre for your egg collection. Skip to the re-grounding stage at the end until you are getting closer to going to theatre. When egg collection is near, move on to the next step of this meditation).

It is almost time to go to theatre and have your eggs collected... this is a good time to explain to your ovaries what is going to happen... tell your eggs they are being collected and they will be safe... not to be scared... that you will always be connected energetically throughout the whole process... if any of your eggs are too small ask them to begin maturing in preparation... if any are too large ask them to slow down and wait for pickup... explain to your eggs that fertilisation will take place soon and ask that they allow that to happen with ease... that they will be stronger once fertilised and a step closer to returning to your body... if you are having a fresh transfer let them know how many will be put back... if they are going to be frozen let them know that they need not be scared... that they are doing an amazing thing for you... and you will wait patiently to see them again in the future... send them a lot of love and gratitude now... spend as long as you need to here until you feel a deep connection with your eggs and your body feels loved and healthy... (again you might want to repeat this a few times leading to your egg pickup. Skip the next stage and go straight to the re-grounding stage. After your egg collection, move on to the next stage of this meditation).

Now that your eggs have been collected, in your mind's eye see them sitting in their petri dish, happy and full... growing as they should... see fertilisation happening with ease... let them know you are still here and waiting for them... remind them they are safe and very wanted... tell them they are loved... if you are having a fresh transfer let them know it's not long now and you will be re-united... if you are having embryos frozen tell them it's safe... that you will send them love the whole time they are frozen... that you will look forward to meeting them again in the future...that even though they are residing outside of your body for a short term, you will always be connected... always a part of you...

If your embryos are being frozen, you might like to do a meditation similar to this throughout the time they are frozen. If you are carrying your own embryos, you might want to move on to the next meditation now. If a surrogate is carrying your embryos for you, skip the next meditation and go to the meditation for surrogacy.

When you are ready, become aware again of the bright colours that have been resting around you, slowly coming back to life, surrounding your body, and bringing your awareness back to your physical body. Become aware of the chair or floor beneath you. You might like to wriggle your toes or your fingers, or your face. And just feel yourself again becoming one with your physical body. Take a nice deep breath in, and when you feel comfortable, that you are safely back in your body, you might like to open your eyes and just take a few moments before you get on with your day.

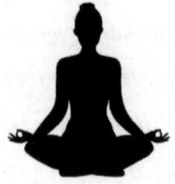

Meditation: for IVF embryo transfer

This meditation focuses on the next stage of IVF when you are having your embryos transferred into your uterus, and is suitable for women carrying their own embryos.

Find yourself a comfortable place to sit or lie down, where you are warm, and your back is supported. Maybe sitting in a chair, or lying on the floor, with a pillow and a blanket. Once you are comfortable, close your eyes and take a nice deep breath in, filling up your lungs with fresh oxygen, all the way down to your tummy. And as you slowly release the breath, feel any tension leaving with it as your body relaxes into the chair or floor beneath you. Again, take another deep breath in, and as the breath turns to leave, feel it picking up your tensions and taking them from your body. Continue to breathe like this for a few moments, breathing in peace and relaxation and breathing out any tension or stress.

Now become aware of a beautiful rainbow light dancing around the top of your head. Swirling around. As it brushes past your skin it picks up and remaining tension dissolving it… and you feel it leave your body. Feel the beautiful vibrant colours of the rainbow, swirl around your head, down over your forehead… across your eyes, your nose, your ears, your cheeks, your mouth and down your jaw. Feel it swirl around your neck and around your shoulders, down both your arms, swirling round your wrists, and your hands and each of your fingers. Feel the rainbow swirling down your trunk… your back, your chest and your sides. Around your buttock and each of your legs, slowly swirling down around past your knees, your calves, your ankles, your feet and each of your toes… As the tension leaves your body feel yourself relaxing heavily into the seat or floor, and the rainbow light just sits softly around you. Relaxing you, keeping you safe and warm, as you continue along this journey.

In your mind's eye bring your attention gently to your uterus now… see your uterus healthy, vibrant… see the endometrial lining thick and welcoming… see the colours vibrant and full of energy… talk softly to your uterus… let it know your embryos are returning soon and the important job it needs to play in accepting and carrying the embryos for you… spend as much time here as you need, gently preparing your uterus and lining…

Now move your focus to your embryos in their petri dish… tell them you are excited to meet them again shortly… that you are ready to welcome them home… that you have your uterus all ready to invite them in… to carry them and support them to grow into the baby you are so excited to meet… see your embryos healthy… calm… ready to be transported back to you…

Now bring your focus to your cervix… let it know that soon it will need to relax and open to allow a catheter to pass through with ease… so your embryos can be returned home… let it know it plays an important role in the process and you are grateful for its help…

You might like to do this meditation a few times in the lead up to your transfer. Skip through to the re-grounding phase until the time of transfer. During the transfer, you might like to do the following step.

It is time for your transfer... allow yourself to relax... the calmer you are, the more relaxed your embryos can be... the more welcoming your body will be to your embryos... as the transfer takes place, in your mind talk to your embryos... say hello... welcome home... I am so excited to see you again... we are ready for you...

Say anything here that feels right for you to establish a loving connection with your embryos. After your transfer, you might like to move on to the next step.

Your embryos are safely back home within your uterus now... see your embryo being welcomed into your endometrial lining... see it supported, happy... growing... healthy... see your lining vibrant with nourishment... talk to your body... tell it how loved it is for the amazing job it is doing... tell it how grateful you are... send love and health to your embryo and to your whole body... stay with this as long as you need to... come back to this meditation often throughout your luteal phase... encouraging your body and sending love every step of the way...

And when you are ready, become aware again of the bright colours that have been resting around you, slowly coming back to life, surrounding your body, and bringing your awareness back to your physical body. Become aware of the chair or floor beneath you. You might like to wriggle your toes or your fingers, or your face. And just feel yourself again becoming one with your physical body. Take a nice deep breath in, and when you feel comfortable, that you are safely back in your body, you might like to open your eyes and just take a few moments before you get on with your day.

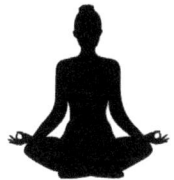

Meditation: for embryos being transferred into a surrogate

This meditation focuses on the next stage of IVF when you are having your embryos transferred into the uterus of your surrogate and is suitable for women not carrying their own embryos.

Find yourself a comfortable place to sit or lie down, where you are warm, and your back is supported. Maybe sitting in a chair, or lying on the floor, with a pillow and a blanket. Once you are comfortable, close your eyes and take a nice deep breath in, filling up your lungs with fresh oxygen, all the way down to your tummy. And as you slowly release the breath, feel any tension leaving with it as your body relaxes into the chair or floor beneath you. Again, take another deep breath in, and as the breath turns to leave, feel it picking up your tensions and taking them from your body. Continue to breathe like this for a few moments, breathing in peace and relaxation and breathing out any tension or stress.

Now become aware of a beautiful rainbow light dancing around the top of your head. Swirling around. As it brushes past your skin it picks up and remaining tension dissolving it... and you feel it leave your body. Feel the beautiful vibrant colours of the rainbow, swirl around your head, down over your forehead... across your eyes, your nose, your ears, your cheeks, your mouth and down your jaw. Feel it swirl around your neck and around your shoulders, down both your arms, swirling round your wrists, and your hands and each of your fingers. Feel the rainbow swirling down your trunk… your back, your chest and your sides. Around your buttock and each of your legs, slowly swirling down around past your knees, your calves, your ankles, your feet and each of your toes… As the tension leaves your body feel yourself relaxing heavily into the seat or floor, and the rainbow light just sits softly around you. Relaxing you, keeping you safe and warm, as you continue along this journey.

In your mind's eye, gently bring your focus to your embryos in their petri dish… explain to them that it is time to be transferred into the uterus of your surrogate… tell them you are excited that a wonderful and generous person is happy to carry them for you… you might like to tell them how you are feeling about not being able to carry them yourself… but remind them they are very loved and very wanted…that you are always connected throughout this process… tell them your surrogate is ready to welcome them… that her uterus is all ready to invite them in… to carry them and support them to grow into the baby you are so excited to meet… see your embryos healthy… calm… ready to be transported to your surrogate… you might like to tell your embryo about your surrogate…

Bring your focus now to your surrogate… in your mind you might like to tell her what a gift she is giving you… send loving energy to her… see it fill her uterus with health and vibrancy… see this beautiful energy extend throughout her whole body… now see a connection from you to her… extend this energetic connection now to your embryos… see a triangular light connect the three of you throughout this process… spend as much time here as you need until you feel the connection… until you see all three of you calm and ready to proceed…

And when you are ready, become aware again of the bright colours that have been resting around you, slowly coming back to life, surrounding your body, and bringing your awareness back to your physical body. Become aware of the chair or floor beneath you. You might like to wriggle your toes or your fingers, or your face. And just feel yourself again becoming one with your physical body. Take a nice deep breath in, and when you feel comfortable, that you are safely back in your body, you might like to open your eyes and just take a few moments before you get on with your day.

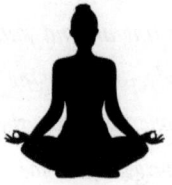

Meditation: for a surrogate

This meditation focuses on the next stage of IVF for a surrogate who is having someone else's embryos transferred into your uterus and is suitable for women acting as a surrogate for someone else.

Find yourself a comfortable place to sit or lie down, where you are warm, and your back is supported. Maybe sitting in a chair, or lying on the floor, with a pillow and a blanket. Once you are comfortable, close your eyes and take a nice deep breath in, filling up your lungs with fresh oxygen, all the way down to your tummy. And as you slowly release the breath, feel any tension leaving with it as your body relaxes into the chair or floor beneath you. Again, take another deep breath in, and as the breath turns to leave, feel it picking up your tensions and taking them from your body. Continue to breathe like this for a few moments, breathing in peace and relaxation and breathing out any tension or stress.

Now become aware of a beautiful rainbow light dancing around the top of your head. Swirling around. As it brushes past your skin it picks up and remaining tension dissolving it... and you feel it leave your body. Feel the beautiful vibrant colours of the rainbow, swirl around your head, down over your forehead... across your eyes, your nose, your ears, your cheeks, your mouth and down your jaw. Feel it swirl around your neck and around your shoulders, down both your arms, swirling round your wrists, and your hands and each of your fingers. Feel the rainbow swirling down your trunk... your back, your chest and your sides. Around your buttock and each of your legs, slowly swirling down around past your knees, your calves, your ankles, your feet and each of your toes... As the tension leaves your body feel yourself relaxing heavily into the seat or floor, and the rainbow light just sits softly around you. Relaxing you, keeping you safe and warm, as you continue along this journey.

In your mind's eye bring your attention gently to your uterus now... see your uterus healthy, vibrant... see the endometrial lining thick and welcoming... see the colours vibrant and full of energy... talk softly to your uterus... let it know the important job it is about to do... the gift it is providing for another person... that this persons embryos are returning soon and the important job it needs to play in accepting and carrying the embryos for her... you might like to tell your uterus about the woman whose embryos you will be carrying... explain why she cannot do this herself... and how you are excited to work together to bring a new life into the world... spend as much time here as you need, gently preparing your uterus and lining...

Now move your focus to your embryos in their petri dish... tell them you are excited to meet them shortly... that you are ready to welcome them... that you have your uterus all ready to invite them in... to carry them and support them to grow into the baby that is so loved and wanted by its mother... see the embryos healthy... calm... ready to be transported to you...

Now bring your focus to your cervix... let it know that soon it will need to relax and open to allow a catheter to pass through with ease... so the embryos can be transferred into your uterus... let it know it plays an important role in the process and *you are grateful for its help...*

Bring your focus now to the woman you are being a surrogate for... in your mind you might like to tell her why you are happy to do this for her... send loving energy to her... now see a connection from you to her... extend this energetic connection now to her embryos... see a triangular light connect the three of you throughout this process... spend as much time here as you need until you feel the connection... until you see all three of you calm and ready to proceed...

You might like to do this meditation a few times in the lead up to the transfer. Skip through to the re-grounding phase until the time of transfer. During the transfer, you might like to do the following step.

It is time for the transfer... allow yourself to relax... the calmer you are, the more relaxed the embryos can be... the more welcoming your body will be to the embryos... as the transfer takes place, in your mind talk to the embryos... say hello... welcome to your temporary home... I am so excited to help bring you to your Mum... we are ready for you...

Say anything here that feels right for you to establish a loving connection with the embryos and to keep them connected to their mum. After your transfer, you might like to move on to the next step.

The embryos are safely home within your uterus now... see the embryo being welcomed into your endometrial lining... see it supported, happy... growing... healthy... see your lining vibrant with nourishment... talk to your body... tell it how loved it is for the amazing job it is doing… tell it how grateful you are… send love and health to your embryo and to your whole body… send this love beyond your body to the Mum whose embryos you are carrying… stay with this as long as you need to… come back to this meditation often throughout your luteal phase… encouraging your body and sending love every step of the way…

And when you are ready, become aware again of the bright colours that have been resting around you, slowly coming back to life, surrounding your body, and bringing your awareness back to your physical body. Become aware of the chair or floor beneath you. You might like to wriggle your toes or your fingers, or your face. And just feel yourself again becoming one with your physical body. Take a nice deep breath in, and when you feel comfortable, that you are safely back in your body, you might like to open your eyes and just take a few moments before you get on with your day.

CHAPTER THIRTEEN
ABUSE AND TRAUMA

"My past will no longer determine my future."

Unfortunately, in my healing work, I see way too many people that have suffered abuse of some kind throughout their lives. Sometimes it is a one-off, perhaps rape, and sometimes it has been for years. It may have been physical, emotional or sexual. Often, this is the cause that comes up for clients that have come to see me for fertility issues.

Abuse can result in a wide variety of emotions that can affect fertility. These include, but are certainly not limited to:

- **Guilt.** Often the victim in abuse is the one left feeling guilty for the abuse. People who never talk about it, or never have the abuse validated by the perpetrator or other authority figure (such as their parents) tend to experience guilt even more profusely than those who have had help in healing the effects of the abuse. The victim may think they 'deserved' it or 'asked for it'. Sometimes they feel like they were 'the other woman' despite never consenting to the abuse, particularly if it was a father-figure who 'chose them' over their mother. In this situation, they not only suffer the physical abuse from the father-figure, but the resentment and anger from the mother. Please refer to chapter nine for more information.

- **Regret.** I doubt you would ever find a survivor of abuse that does not wish it hadn't happened. They may feel a lot of regret for being in the wrong place at the wrong time, for wishing they'd dressed differently, acted differently, been less attractive. They may regret walking home alone or leaving work after dark. They might regret befriending the person that abused them, or for not getting help, or for not standing up for themselves. Regret is often a feeling that coincides with feeling defeated.

- **Fear.** There can be a deep held fear that what happened to you could happen to your child, and who would want to bring a child into that sort of world? If you cannot protect yourself, how can you protect your child? If you do become pregnant to the perpetrator, how could you look at your baby's face every day and not be reminded of the abuse? So, you may pray continuously not to get pregnant, or you may have had to have an abortion in the past. This creates a whole other level to fertility issues. See the issue on miscarriage, stillborn and abortion in chapter sixteen.

- **Disgust.** This is a common feeling for victims of abuse. Disgust for attracting the unwanted attention in the first place, disgust for allowing it to happen. Often when there is abuse, the physical body displays the physical response of enjoyment. This can create a level of disgust for having an enjoyable physical response, even though enjoyment is a normal response to the physical stimuli.

- **Anger.** A very common reaction to abuse is to feel anger. In a lot of ways anger is a safer emotion than others, it is easier to express and feel. Anger at the perpetrator, anger at yourself, anger at those around for not seeing or helping. Left unresolved, anger can present as various physical ailments in the body. It can also affect relationships, careers and every other aspect of your life.

- **Acceptance.** We are talking mentally and physically. While you may have had counselling and feel you have 'moved on' from the abuse, sometimes your body continues to 'hold the abuse' and this can lead to physical pain and illness. I often work on clients with Forensic Healing, and their abuse comes up as the cause of their issue, and they will tell me, 'But, I already dealt with this!' and they did mentally, but their body needs to release it as well, and energy healing is a great way to do this.

- **Weight issues.** Often people who have experienced abuse carry extra weight as a protective mechanism, for example they may believe if they are fat no one will look at them 'in that way' or 'want to have sex with them'. Carrying extra weight impacts fertility, so being able to heal from abuse may also help with weight issues, and therefore fertility issues.

Men who have suffered abuse may have issues around infertility also for all of the above reasons. They may also find it difficult to be intimate with another person. It can also raise all sorts of issues for them regarding if they can be a good parent, if they can protect their child, and if they actually want to bring a child into a world where such horrific things can happen. It is not as socially acceptable for men to discuss their abuse as it is for women. This statement isn't to cause offence or start an argument, but it has been my observation that the man that admits to being sexually abused is often looked at and treated very differently to the woman who was sexually abused. Hopefully in time, it will become easier for men to discuss abuse, so they can grieve and heal and live a happy and healthy life.

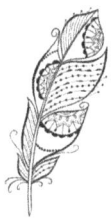

Journaling: for abuse therapy

Have you been a victim of abuse at any stage in your life? If it feels safe to do so, please write about this experience now. Writing is an effective way of *starting* the emotional healing process. How did you felt during and after, your thoughts and reactions at the time, what you told yourself to cope? Writing this down will help you heal the negative feelings. If you haven't already, it is highly likely you will need professional help to work through your experience, and I would encourage you to seek this help.

CHAPTER FOURTEEN
CULTURAL CONSIDERATIONS

"I can have a baby while respecting my culture and heritage."

As I sit here in Australia writing this, I can choose who I marry. I can get married and divorced as I see fit. I can decide the best way for me to juggle having a family and a career. It's all up to me. Yes, my family and friends have opinions on what I do, but ultimately, I get to decide how I live my life.

This isn't the case in many cultures. I am certainly not an expert on cultural relationships, so this chapter is based on conversations I have had and observations I have made. It will not apply to every culture or every person, but it may provide some insight.

In some cultures, the bride and groom are chosen by the parents. An advertisement goes in the paper, advertising a potential bride or groom, and the parents consider which advertisements to respond to. The bride's parents will meet with the groom and his family, to decide if their children are suited to each other. Once the decision is made this is a good fit, the bride will meet the groom. They will generally meet a few times before getting married.

Once married, the bride would traditionally move into the groom's family home. In a culture where family is incredibly important, this would be a big transition for the bride leaving her family and joining a new family she barely knows. There is a lot of pressure to be a good daughter-in-law and wife.

Sex is generally not openly discussed at any stage of the woman's life. The bride has a basic understanding of what sex is, but it is not a topic that is freely explored, questions are not asked, and cycles are not well explained. Sex is essentially a chore that neither partner particularly enjoys in most marriages. There is usually no foreplay and no intimacy.

There is a lot of pressure to start a family at this point. From what I've been told, if a pregnancy hasn't occurred within six months, questions will be asked and a lot of pressure is applied. This pressure is not just from the groom and his parents, but aunties, grandparents, neighbours and everyone has an opinion and can voice it freely. If time goes on and the woman cannot get pregnant, there is also the risk the groom will be told to divorce his wife and find a new bride who can provide children. Once divorced for being infertile, there is little chance of the woman finding a new husband that would want her. If the bride's family has paid a lot of money towards the union, this can create a lot of conflict within the bride's family also.

- There is a lot of pressure and stress. And, guess what the worst thing for the reproductive cycle functioning well is? Stress.
- There are many aspects to be considered when it comes to cultural infertility.
- Moving away from the family home and known support systems. This can be compounded if the couple move to another country, which is also often the case. The bride finds herself in a place where she knows no one, barely knows her husband, and doesn't speak the language in order to make new friendships and build new support systems.

- There is a huge amount of pressure to conceive and quickly, and preferably with a son to carry on the family name.
- There is no understanding of the menstrual cycle and reproductive systems, so no way of knowing when the fertile time of the month is.
- Sex is widely misunderstood and not generally enjoyed. It is a chore that needs to be done and probably isn't done frequently, therefore likely missing the fertile window month-after-month.
- The pressure to conceive and the fear of not being able to do this, compounded by the fact the husband may replace the wife if it doesn't happen, results in an incredible amount of stress on the body.

I have been asked questions that seem ridiculous to someone with a basic understanding of the reproductive system, but it makes perfect sense when someone has no knowledge of how the body works, especially when it comes to fertility. Observations like the wife rolls over too often in bed when asleep, is that why she cannot get pregnant? Questions like she sits at a computer all day at work, does that squash the ovaries and stop them working? Interestingly, and this isn't a judgement but merely another observation, there is rarely any question about the man's sperm quality, which is often not tested, or their behaviours and actions that affect fertility. The assumption is most often that the issue lies with the woman. It does not generally even occur to the man that he may be the issue.

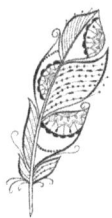

Journaling: for cultural awareness

1. What cultural considerations do you need to respect and adhere to?

2. Can you see any correlation with not becoming pregnant and the ideas outlined above?

CHAPTER FIFTEEN
SECONDARY INFERTILITY

"I am deserving of more than one child."

Sometimes you conceive your first baby easily and naturally and then you have a lot of difficulty achieving pregnancy again. This is called secondary infertility and is common.

There are some obvious reasons for this happening, such as already having a child means you are busier, probably tired, there is less time for intercourse with your partner, and potentially no time when ovulation is actually happening.

Even when people track their cycles and ensure they have intercourse at ovulation time pregnancy may still not occur.

Some of the emotional issues I have witnessed in relation to this include:

'I already have a child, I should just be grateful for what I have.'

Okay, this could be true, and I am sure you are incredibly grateful for the child you already have. However, that doesn't mean you are not 'entitled' or 'worthy' of having a second or third child. It doesn't make it hurt any less when the pregnancy doesn't occur month after month. And you don't need to feel guilty for being able to have more than one child. There isn't a certain number of babies available in the world, and you are not selfish for taking an extra one out of the bag that someone else could have had. You having another baby does not take the opportunity away from another person, so please address any feelings of guilt or selfishness you may be experiencing.

'I can barely keep up with the child I have, how could I manage another?'

Very few people in this day and age feel as though they are doing a great job as a parent, in my experience. There is more expectation to return to work, to manage the household efficiently and to contribute to the financial needs of the family. This can be tiring and overwhelming and is a legitimate question. If you are facing this issue, it might be time for a heart-to-heart with your significant other, if you have one, or other support networks to see what changes you can put in place to make having another child a viable and enjoyable option.

'I am older now, so of course it will be harder.'

It is true that as we get older, our fertility decreases. We have fewer eggs and they are often of lesser quality. In this instance it might be worthwhile seeking further help or investigations earlier. Ensuring you are as fit and healthy as possible can help, maintain a healthy weight and exercise regime, get plenty of sleep and manage your stress.

Having had a child previously is a good indicator of being successful with a second pregnancy.

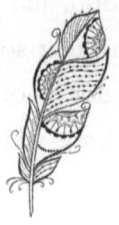

Journaling: shifting perspectives for baby 2

Explore the following questions and note any changes you can make to optimise your chances of a successful pregnancy. Consider how your life is different now to when you had your first baby.

1. You are obviously older, but what other factors are playing a role?
2. What is your weight, diet and exercise regime like compared to last time?
3. Are you with the same partner, if so, has anything changed with him or his health?
4. Are your cycles still the same, or are they changing?
5. How are your stress levels, your sleep patterns?

CHAPTER SIXTEEN
FERTILITY AFTER MISCARRIAGE, ABORTION OR A STILLBORN

"I give myself permission to grieve my loss and to move on when I'm ready."

Losing a baby is one of the most difficult things a person will ever go through. Even if you've only known you're pregnant for a short time, there is a good chance you have been planning that baby's life from the minute you knew you were pregnant. Wondering about the gender of the baby, carefully selecting names, imagining how they will look, the funny little quirks of their personality. So, the loss of a pregnancy at any stage can be heartbreaking. Sadly, one in six pregnancies result in a miscarriage before the age of 20 weeks (IVFA). Often, we are told, particularly with early pregnancy loss, that 'it wasn't even a baby yet', that you can 'simply have another one'. We are expected to get over it quickly and effortlessly.

Often when there is an early pregnancy loss, it indicates an issue with the foetus, that perhaps chromosomally there was something wrong that was incompatible with life. Sometimes testing can be done to identify the cause, which may give you some closure and alleviate future fears of another loss. However, often you won't know why, and you will move on without an answer and possibly some fears and unresolved grief.

What I am suggesting is you take the time to grieve your loss. A loss at any stage is still a loss, and you are allowed to feel sad, or angry, or whatever emotion you are feeling. You might not feel any of these things, you might find it easy to accept the loss and plan for your future, and this is fine too. But give yourself the space and time to feel whatever you feel, because it will be unique for you. Addressing any emotions and feelings at the time of the loss may save you future heartache also.

In the event of a miscarriage, you may need to 'clear the space in the womb'. This may sound strange and a little far-fetched, but is it possible that energetically your uterus is already being filled by the baby you lost. I have been told by women that have had miscarriages, that they feel as though they are 'cheating' on their lost baby by wanting another. My belief of our world, which may be controversial for some but hopefully comforting for others, is that we are all spiritual beings, we come here to fulfil a destiny or learn a lesson, and we return to where we came from, as a spiritual being, loved unconditionally when our time here is done. I often think when a child is here for only a short time, that perhaps they chose that journey to assist you on yours. A child that has left this world will not hold any blame or anger towards you. These are human emotions that pass when one returns to be a spiritual being.

Having a stillborn is different to a miscarriage in the sense you gave birth to your child. The loss will affect your body and emotions in a different way. When you have had a stillborn you have seen your child, you gave birth to your child, and you have had to bury your child. I have been told by women that have had a stillborn, or lost a child when they were older, that if they had planned on a certain number of children, they feel like they are doing the wrong thing by not counting the deceased child in that number. My thoughts are that child would want their parents to be happy, so it is okay to let yourself out of that contract you made with yourself, if it feels like the right thing to do. Ask the child you lost to help you make the best decisions for you, to send you the baby that is the best fit for your family, and to watch over the baby during pregnancy and life. Your child will know how loved and wanted they were, they won't resent you for wanting to have another child. It is not to replace them, but to complete your family.

Having an abortion can raise many other issues and emotions. The woman who made the choice that was right for her and felt okay with it is less likely to experience infertility and other health issues after an abortion, than the woman who felt forced into it, and the abortion was not what she wanted. I have seen clients that also felt they made the right decision at the time for them or convinced themselves it was their only option and they were okay with it, only to find down the track that they regretted it or had health issues such as infertility and associated ailments, that stem from the abortion. Unresolved grief, loss, anger or resentment will generally appear somewhere in the body at some point if not addressed and processed. If you have had an abortion, regardless if you felt okay with it or not, I would urge you to do the activity below. Sometimes we are not even aware that energetically our body is holding on to something, even if our mind has convinced us we are okay.

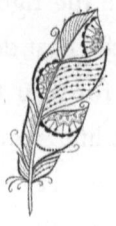

Journaling: to heal the womb

1. **Miscarriage.** A simple technique is to give yourself time when you won't be interrupted to sit quietly and bring your attention to your uterus. If you can, visualise your lost baby. This may be as a baby, as a colour, or simply as a feeling within your uterus. Out loud or in your head, say all of the things you would have liked to have said to that baby. That you loved it, how much you wanted it, how much you still want it. Tell it it's okay to move on now and ask for its assistance and protection for any future babies.

2. **Stillborn.** You can use the same technique as above, but this time visualise holding the baby in your arms to say your goodbyes, instead of in the uterus.

3. **Abortion.** In the event of an abortion, whether you were okay with the decision or not, you can use the above technique to help yourself and your body let go of the emotions and move on. In this instance, you might like to tell your child your reasons for the abortion, knowing they are now a spiritual being and can understand this from that perspective, not that of a small child. You might like to explain why you made the decision, and that even though perhaps it is still affecting you now, you need to find peace with it, so you can move on.

4. Ask the baby you lost for assistance to bring another healthy baby into the world for you to love and cherish.

If you need further help with this, and if you need counselling to help you address these emotions, I would urge you to do so.

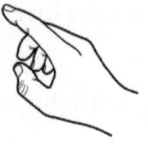

Tapping Script 4: for trying for a baby after having lost one

Often there are mixed feelings when trying for a baby after having lost one. Some people take relief from the fact they know they can get pregnant as sometimes that is a big step forward. Some people hold fear that if they lost one already perhaps that will continue, or maybe there was something wrong with their baby that caused the loss and that could continue. Sometimes people feel guilt for wanting a new pregnancy when they lost one. Your reactions and emotions could vary greatly during this time and may change from one minute to the next. That is the beauty of tapping, it is versatile, and you can use it as often as you need to as your emotions change. Some of the points below may not apply to you, it's unlikely you will feel all of these things at any one time, so please use the parts that apply to you and change or leave out the ones that don't. Your previous loss may have been due to miscarriage, stillborn, abortion or the loss of a child after he or she was born, which will also impact how you feel and how the tapping applies to you. For this purpose of this script I will simply refer to the loss as a loss, but you can make it specific to your circumstances if you find that helpful.

The karate point (KP): Even though I lost my baby,
I love and accept myself deeply and completely.
KP: Even though I want another baby,

I love and accept myself deeply and completely.

KP: Even though I want another baby after already losing one,

I love and accept myself deeply and completely.

Inner Eye (IE): I lost my baby

Outer Eye (OE): that hurts

Under Eye (UE): I had hoped to hold my bay in my arms

Under Nose (UN): to watch her/him grow up

Under Mouth (UM): and that future has been taken away from me

Collarbone (CB) *use fist*: I lost my baby

Under Arm (UA) *use hand*: and that hurts

Top of the head (TH): but I still want all of those things

IE: I want to try again

OE: I want another chance

UE: but I lost one

UN: and I might lose another one

UM: and that's a painful thought

CB: it hurts to have lost one

UA: it hurts to know I may lose another

TH: I'm not sure how much hurt I can take

IE: was there something wrong with my baby?

OE: is that why I lost him/her?

UE: if so, what's to say it won't keep happening?

UN: I could keep losing them

UM: there might be something wrong with all of them

CB: something wrong with me

UA: there's so much fear

TH: I don't know what's going to happen

IE: is it wrong to want another one?

OE: I can't replace the one I lost

UE: is it wrong to want to try?

UN: I feel guilty because I want to

UM: guilty and scared

CB: guilty and angry

UA: why did I have to go through this?

TH: wasn't infertility painful enough already?

Keep going as long as you need to, being as specific to your circumstances and feelings as you can be.

IE: it's okay to keep trying

OE: that baby wasn't ready to come into the world

UE: but I am allowed to keep trying

UN: perhaps there was something wrong

UM: but that doesn't mean the next one won't be healthy

CB: I am choosing to trust that it's safe to keep trying

UA: so, I let go of any guilt I'm holding on to

TH: I let go of the anger and the hurt

IE: I will look for the positives

OE: if I was pregnant once I can be pregnant again

UE: my body is learning what to do

UN: it is safe to hope I will bring a healthy baby in to the world

UM: I trust in the process

CB: I am allowed to want a baby

UA: even though I lost one

TH: it is safe to keep trying.

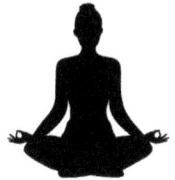

Meditation: for previous miscarriages

Experiencing a miscarriage is difficult. From the minute you know you are pregnant, you start to plan the life of that child. You might consider names, wonder if it will be a boy or a girl, imagine announcing their arrival to your friends and family, telling your partner you are pregnant. When a miscarriage happens, it can feel like the end of those dreams, and it's not always easy to let that go and move on to trying again. This meditation focuses on clearing the space where that baby once was and preparing the space for a new pregnancy. This meditation is suitable for any woman that has experienced a miscarriage.

Take notice of your breath. Take a deep breath in for 5, all the way down to your abdomen. Hold it for a moment… then slowly release the breath as you count to 5. Hold again and then breathe in again… counting to five… continue to breathe this way. As you breathe in, imagine a clear crystal rod from your crown chakra on the top of your head, extending down to your root chakra at the base of your spine. See the crystal rod changing colour with your breath as you relax, deeper and deeper. Violet…indigo…blue at the throat…green…yellow…passing your navel…orange…red…

Allow your mind to clear of all other thoughts. Let any fears… worries and tension dissolve from your body… gently floating out of the top of your head. Now see a glass box in your mind's eye. In this box is a bright flickering candle. Focus on the candle, as you allow yourself to be still. This is your time just to be. Silent... Still. Use the energy of the candle to re-charge your tired mind and body. Let the warm glow refresh you. Know that when life brings you fear or worry, you can focus on the candle and welcome stillness...

When you are ready let your focus shift from the candle to your tummy... going within... and as you look deep within your tummy you see the spirit of the baby that was once living there... the spirit is content, unaware he or she should have moved on... as you look lovingly at the beautiful little being that was yours, allow any feelings or emotions to come... there is no judgement here... no right way to feel... whatever you feel is perfectly okay and normal... spend as much time here as you need with this little being... you might like to tell him or her what your dreams for them had been... how much you loved them and wanted them... tell them you are sorry they couldn't stay with you... offer forgiveness for them leaving and ask for forgiveness for any fears you may have about what went wrong... forgive yourself for any judgements you hold towards yourself now... sending only love to yourself from this point forward... you might like to ask your little spirit baby if he or she has any messages for you... if it feels right to do so, you might like to ask this being if it will help you to conceive again, to bring you a new baby, and to watch over this baby as it grows and develops into a healthy baby... when you are ready, tell this beautiful little being it is time to move on... it's okay to return home... as you return your focus to the candle in your mind's eye, see it glow brighter and brighter and know your baby is passing through that light and returning home to where it belongs... and this place can be any place that feels right for you...

When you are ready, imagine the glow of the candle now moving towards your tummy… filling the space with a beautiful clearing and healing light… see the light move to any part of your uterus that needs healing… until all that is left is a fresh, clear space that is ready to welcome a pregnancy… spend as much time as you need here, preparing the space with love and healing energy…

When you are ready, bring your awareness back to your breathing… Take a deep breath in … 1,2,3,4,5. Hold it for a moment… Now release it slowly for 5… Again, holding at the end of the exhale. Now focus again on the crystal rod extending from your base chakra to your crown chakra. Starting at the base, imagine red light going to your feet, legs, hips and spine. See orange light coming up your abdomen… turning to yellow. Green light fills your heart… your lungs. Feel blue light going up to your throat… your neck and into your jaw. Indigo light awakens your ears… your eyes and nose. Now let a violet light bring sensation back to your whole body as it protectively wraps around you… and open your eyes when you are ready.

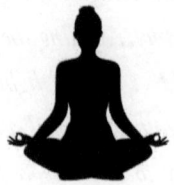

Meditation: for previous abortions

Making the decision to have an abortion is not always an easy one. Sometimes neither option feels right, but you have to make the best decision for you based on the circumstances at the time. I have worked with women that have had abortions and have experienced seemingly unrelated health issues later in life, which is the body's way of expressing the grief they may not have been able to express at the time. Sometimes there is an element of guilt, or anger. This meditation focuses on clearing the space where that baby once was and preparing the space for a new pregnancy. This meditation is suitable for any woman that has experienced an abortion, regardless if you felt it was the right option for you or not at the time.

> *Take notice of your breath. Take a deep breath in for 5, all the way down to your abdomen. Hold it for a moment... then slowly release the breath as you count to 5. Hold again and then breathe in again... counting to five... continue to breathe this way. As you breathe in, imagine a clear crystal rod from your crown chakra on the top of your head, extending down to your root chakra at the base of your spine. See the crystal rod changing colour with your breath as you relax, deeper and deeper. Violet...indigo...blue at the throat...green...yellow...passing your navel...orange...red...*
>
> *Allow your mind to clear of all other thoughts. Let any*

fears... worries and tension dissolve from your body... gently floating out of the top of your head. Now see a glass box in your mind's eye. In this box is a bright flickering candle. Focus on the candle, as you allow yourself to be still. This is your time just to be. Silent... Still. Use the energy of the candle to re-charge your tired mind and body. Let the warm glow refresh you. Know that when life brings you fear or worry, you can focus on the candle and welcome stillness...

When you are ready let your focus shift from the candle to your tummy... going within... and as you look deep within your tummy you see the spirit of the baby that was once living there... the spirit is content, unaware he or she should have moved on... as you look lovingly at the beautiful little being that was yours, allow any feelings or emotions to come... there is no judgement here... no right way to feel... whatever you feel is perfectly okay and normal... spend as much time here as you need with this little being... you might like to tell him or her your reasons for having the abortion... how you felt about it then... ow you feel about it now... tell them you are sorry they couldn't stay with you... ask for forgiveness for any fears you may have had then or now... forgive yourself for any judgements you hold towards yourself now... sending only love to yourself from this point forward... you might like to ask your little spirit baby if he or she has any messages for you... if it feels right to do so, you might like to ask this being if it will help you to conceive again, to bring you a new baby, and to watch over this baby as it grows and develops into a healthy baby, knowing there is no judgement from this Divine being... only love, forgiveness and understanding... when you are ready, tell this beautiful little being it is time to move on... it's okay to return home... as you return your focus to the candle in your mind's eye, see it glow brighter and brighter and know your baby is passing through that light and returning home to where it belongs... to a place that feels right for you...

When you are ready, imagine the glow of the candle now moving towards your tummy... filling the space with a beautiful clearing and healing light... see the light move to any part of your uterus that needs healing... until all that is left is a fresh, clear space that is ready to welcome a pregnancy... spend as much time as you need here, preparing the space with love and healing energy...

When you are ready, bring your awareness back to your breathing... Take a deep breath in... 1,2,3,4,5. Hold it for a moment... Now release it slowly for 5... Again, holding at the end of the exhale. Now focus again on the crystal rod extending from your base chakra to your crown chakra. Starting at the base, imagine red light going to your feet, legs, hips and spine. See orange light coming up your abdomen... turning to yellow. Green light fills your heart... your lungs. Feel blue light going up to your throat... your neck and into your jaw. Indigo light awakens your ears... your eyes and nose. Now let a violet light bring sensation back to your whole body as it protectively wraps around you... and open your eyes when you are ready.

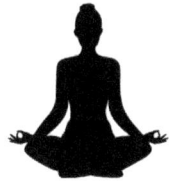

Meditation: for a previous stillborn

Having a stillborn baby is an incredibly difficult experience. Sometimes you know during the pregnancy that your child has passed, or it might be that you found out once they were born. It's important to give yourself time to grieve your loss, knowing the loss is a very real and significant one, regardless of how far into your pregnancy you were. It's not always easy to let that child go in these circumstances and move on to trying again. I've been told it feels like you are 'cheating' on the previous baby, or that you are trying to replace it. This meditation focuses on healing any judgements you hold around this and helps to prepare a space for a new pregnancy. This meditation is suitable for any woman that has experienced a stillborn.

Take notice of your breath. Take a deep breath in for 5, all the way down to your abdomen. Hold it for a moment… then slowly release the breath as you count to 5. Hold again and then breathe in again… counting to five… continue to breathe this way. As you breathe in, imagine a clear crystal rod from your crown chakra on the top of your head, extending down to your root chakra at the base of your spine. See the crystal rod changing colour with your breath as you relax, deeper and deeper. Violet…indigo…blue at the throat…green…yellow…passing your navel…orange…red…

Allow your mind to clear of all other thoughts. Let any

fears… worries and tension dissolve from your body… gently floating out of the top of your head. Now see a glass box in your mind's eye. In this box is a bright flickering candle. Focus on the candle, as you allow yourself to be still. This is your time just to be. Silent… Still. Use the energy of the candle to re-charge your tired mind and body. Let the warm glow refresh you. Know that when life brings you fear or worry, you can focus on the candle and welcome stillness…

When you are ready let your focus shift from the candle to your arms that once held your baby for a brief time. As you look at your arms, you see yourself cradling the spirit of the baby that was once there… the spirit baby is content, unaware he or she should have moved on… as you look lovingly at the beautiful little being that was yours, allow any feelings or emotions to come… there is no judgement here… no right way to feel… whatever you feel is perfectly okay and normal… spend as much time here as you need with this little being… you might like to tell him or her what your dreams for them had been… how much you loved them and wanted them… tell them you are sorry they couldn't stay with you…offer forgiveness for them leaving and ask for forgiveness for any fears you may have about what went wrong… forgive yourself for any judgements you hold towards yourself now… sending only love to yourself from this point forward… you might like to ask your little spirit baby if he or she has any messages for you… if it feels right to do so, you might like to ask this being if it will help you to conceive again, to bring you a baby, and to watch over his or her sibling as it grows and develops into a healthy baby… when you are ready, tell this beautiful little being it is time to move on… it's okay to return home… as you return your focus to the candle in your mind's eye, see it glow brighter and brighter and know your baby is passing through that light and returning home to where it belongs... to a place that feels right for you...

When you are ready, imagine the glow of the candle now moving towards your tummy... filling the space with a beautiful clearing and healing light... see the light move to any part of your uterus that needs healing... until all that is left is a fresh, clear space that is ready to welcome a pregnancy... spend as much time as you need here, preparing the space with love and healing energy...

When you are ready, bring your awareness back to your breathing... Take a deep breath in... 1,2,3,4,5. Hold it for a moment... Now release it slowly for 5... Again, holding at the end of the exhale. Now focus again on the crystal rod extending from your base chakra to your crown chakra. Starting at the base, imagine red light going to your feet, legs, hips and spine. See orange light coming up your abdomen... turning to yellow. Green light fills your heart... your lungs. Feel blue light going up to your throat... your neck and into your jaw. Indigo light awakens your ears... your eyes and nose. Now let a violet light bring sensation back to your whole body as it protectively wraps around you... and open your eyes when you are ready.

CHAPTER SEVENTEEN
WHAT ABOUT THE MEN

"I am an equal partner in our fertility journey."

While this book is mostly focusing on women, and while many of the chapters and activities can be applied to the man in your life also, I thought I should also consider some of the most common issues for men when looking at infertility.

Traditionally, men are considered manly. They provide for the family, they are strong, and they can breed. So, finding out that sperm quality is not great for a man may not only be a big shock, but also a knock to their self-confidence and to the beliefs they held about themselves. I don't say this to sound condescending, although I'm aware it could be taken this way, but I can assure you it's not my intention.

Sperm problems can be a result of many different factors. Depending on the medical cause—if one is found—treatments will vary. You can help yourself by maintaining a healthy diet, regular exercise, quitting smoking, and avoiding drugs such as steroid use.

According to Inna Segal, a problem with the testes can result from a man feeling threatened, exposed and insecure, holding on to guilt, shame, anger, and difficulty forgiving and moving on. If the infertility is due to an issue with the penis, this can be a result of a lack of belief in self, fear of intimacy, feelings of rejection, anger, guilt or victimisation.

If you find yourself looking for excuses to not have sex with your partner, or deliberately avoiding the topic, it might be time to have an honest think about if you are actually wanting to father a child? You may question if this is the right time or the right partner. You may be worried about finances, about it affecting your relationship or lifestyle, or your ability to be a good father depending on your history and upbringing. Now would be a good time to review these topics and decide the way forward. I would encourage you to discuss this with your partner, if you are both wanting something different out of life, then a child is not the best way forward, and while it's difficult, it is much better for both of you to decide this before bringing a baby into the world.

I was talking to a couple that had lost their second child at almost full term. They didn't receive an explanation for the loss, and they struggled to come to terms with it. It resulted in a lot of anxiety and heartbreak for both of them. I'll introduce them under fictitious names, Katie and Jack, for the purpose of this chapter. When Katie felt ready to try again, a pregnancy just didn't happen. She underwent tests and saw fertility specialists, but no cause was found. Eventually, the doctor took her husband Jack aside and asked him how he was feeling about it all. Jack admitted he was terrified of watching his wife go through the pain of another loss. He wanted another child, but not at the cost of his wife's health and well-being. I believe this couple was so lucky to have such a switched-on doctor, who encouraged Jack to go home and talk through his fears and feelings with Katie. This brought them closer as a couple, and they were able to better support each other though the pregnancy that resulted soon after, and they now have a healthy baby.

Our mind, including our beliefs and fears, really does have a strong influence over our physical health. There is a lot of research and evidence to support this which is easy to find if you are needing convincing. Even if you are not fully convinced, where's the harm in exploring your beliefs and fears and seeing if there is a correlation between that and your fertility? Having an honest conversation with yourself, your partner, or a counsellor may be the key to achieving a pregnancy.

On a final note, I have also seen women go through months of tests and tracking, to find out their husband has had a vasectomy and either didn't know how to tell their partner or chose not to. Please don't do this. Honesty, while sometimes difficult, is really important for a healthy relationship, and you need to have a healthy relationship if you are going to bring a child into the world.

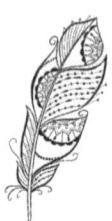

Journaling: for him

Do you have a physical issue affecting your fertility that you know of? If so, do the explanations above reflect your situation or feelings? Are there health and lifestyle change you need to make? Do you want to be a Dad? Did the questions above raise any issues or concerns for you?

CHAPTER EIGHTEEN
WHAT IF I'M NO LONGER INFERTILE?

"It is okay for me to feel a range of emotions now I'm pregnant."

What about once you're pregnant?

So much focus is on the process of trying to become pregnant, that sometimes we can become defined by our infertility. So, once you are pregnant and no longer infertile, who are you? What about the support groups and all the friends you've made that are still infertile? How do those friendships survive if they are now feeling resentment towards you for achieving what they so desperately want? Conversations can become stilted, uncomfortable.

I spoke to a woman that was going through the infertility journey at the same time as her closest friend. When she finally became pregnant, her friend was so angry she stopped talking to her altogether. She felt so much guilt for being pregnant. Sadly within a few weeks she lost her baby. The last I heard, her friend had finally achieved a pregnancy, but she was still trying after her loss and the friendship was still not repaired.

Jealousy can be an incredibly difficult feeling to manage, and if steps aren't taken to address it, jealousy can change who you are, it can stop you from being able to feel happiness for others, and it can change your relationships forever. Do the activities at the end of this chapter to gain perspective in this situation and hopefully save any friendships that might otherwise become strained during the infertility process.

Another issue you may face once pregnancy is achieved is how you balance the fear that it might be too good to be true, that it may not *stay* with being positive, and enjoying the pregnancy? I spoke to one girl that said she had to hold on firmly to the fear of losing the pregnancy, because if she let that go, she was sure she would lose the pregnancy and the pain of that loss would be too much to bear. It felt safer to spend nine months worrying than to relax and enjoy it.

Another girl with a history of a stillborn, told me she was so sure something would go wrong during this new pregnancy that even after she delivered a healthy baby, she couldn't relax and enjoy her. She was quite sure that if she did, something would happen to her baby, something would go wrong. She could not let her guard down even for a moment. As we talked through it, it made sense to her why she felt the way she did given her previous stillborn, and I gave her tools such as tapping to try and help with the anxiety. She was also in close contact with medical care.

Unfortunately, it is human nature to believe the worst rather than hope for the best. It feels like the safer option to expect the worst and have it happen, as opposed to hoping for the best and being let down.

Sometimes after the baby is born, it isn't at all how you imagined it would be. The sleepless nights take a toll, the friends you may have had previously are still going with their infertility journey and for various reasons may not be around as much. They might be busy with their fertility appointments, appointments that once occupied your days but are now no longer necessary. It might be simply too painful for them to be around you and your baby. I would strongly urge anyone that has been infertile but is now a mum or soon to be, to seek counselling to talk through any of these issues that come up if needed. It is a huge change in life, one you thought you might never have, and there will be a whole array of emotions, mixed in with hormones and sleep deprivation. Don't ever feel you can't get help if you need it.

One girl said to me that after going through IVF for her baby she felt she couldn't complain about the things other mothers complained about because she'd gone through so much to get her child. She felt guilty if she complained she was tired, or if she needed some time out. Not only was her journey to becoming a mum different to her friends, but her motherhood journey also felt very different.

If your whole focus is and has been for some time on actually getting pregnant, once you become pregnant you may feel a little lost in who you are and how your life now looks. If you've been having continuous visits to a fertility clinic and constant tests and communication with your nurse, you might feel a little abandoned once this is no longer part of your life. Your visits will likely stop by the time you reach 12 weeks of pregnancy, and this also means the close monitoring will stop. This can raise a lot of concerns about how your baby is travelling, if it is okay, if everything is happening as it should be. Every minor pain or sensation could send you into a panic. This is where a reliable pregnancy book is invaluable. Side note: Dr Google will likely cause you more concerns. Once you are booked into an ante-natal clinic or seeing a specialist, find out what help is available to you. Who can you ring if you are worried, what support is readily accessible? Fear can feed on itself and bring you a lot of stress, so if you know these things in advance, you will most likely find you don't have to use them too often.

Also finding a trusted source that has been through it, such as, your mother, a friend, an aunty, grandma, that is a calming influence, may also be helpful.

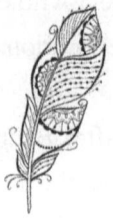

Journaling: writing for a positive pregnancy

1. How would or do you feel when someone close to you becomes pregnant while you are going through infertility? Does this change your relationship with them in any way?

2. If you were to become pregnant, how would you want your friends to react and treat you? Is this different to what you wrote in question one?

3. I want you to write two letters. The first is to the friend who has achieved a pregnancy while you are still trying. It can be a made-up friend if need be, you won't be sending the letter either way. Talk about how you feel and what you are finding difficult. Then talk about how you want to be, how you want your friendship to be, and how you are going to choose to feel and react in this scenario. The second letter is from you once you have achieved a pregnancy to a friend wo is still going through infertility. Repeat the process from the first letter but from this different perspective. Do these two letters give you some insight into both perspectives? Does it help to address some of the feelings that came up for you? Are there areas of your life you can apply what you have now learned?

4. Have you thought much about life after your infertility?

How pregnancy might be for you, how motherhood will be? It is worth considering these things and planning how you will find support during these stages if needed.

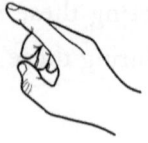

Tapping Script 5: for once you are pregnant

You might be wondering why there would be a need for tapping once you are pregnant. I mean that is the end goal, right? You must be over the moon, excited and elated. And you probably are all of those things. But often in addition to feeling very happy and grateful, there is an element of fear. After waiting so long and trying so hard, what if something goes wrong now? What if you lose the baby, or what if there's something wrong with it. What if you're not a good parent after all and there was a reason you weren't getting pregnant? What if your friends are jealous or resentful of you now you are pregnant and they're not your friends anymore. Who are you now you are not infertile? This could be a time of great joy and confusion. The tapping script is very general as you may be experiencing a few or many of the issues outlined. Use the ones you need to, skip over the ones you don't or change the words to suit your specific circumstances and feelings. Know it's okay to feel any emotions you are feeling. Nothing is right or wrong, it just is.

> The karate point (KP): Even though I am so excited and grateful to be pregnant I am also quite terrified, but
> I love and accept myself deeply and completely.
> KP: Even though I'm scared something will go wrong,

I love and accept myself deeply and completely.

KP: Even though I'm worried my friends won't like me anymore,

I love and accept myself deeply and completely.

Inner Eye (IE): I am so excited to be pregnant finally

Outer Eye (OE): but if I'm honest I'm also scared

Under Eye (UE): it took so long to get pregnant

Under Nose (UN): what if it doesn't stay?

Under Mouth (UM): what if there's something wrong with it?

Collarbone (CB) *use fist*: am I tempting fate trying to make this happen

Under Arm (UA) *use hand*: maybe nature knew best

Top of the head (TH): what if it all goes wrong?

IE: I can't relax and enjoy it

OE: because I'm worried I'll jinx myself

UE: if I let my guard down something will go wrong

UN: it's all too good to be true

UM: what if I mess it up?

CB: what if I do something wrong?

UA: I couldn't cope to lose it now

TH: it would hurt too much

IE: what will my friends say?

OE: they are still infertile

UE: will they hate me?

UN: will they be jealous?

UM: should I tell them?

CB: is it rubbing it in their face if I tell them?

UA: is it wrong to not tell them when we've shared this journey together so far?

TH: I wish they were pregnant too

IE: what if all my friends disown me?

OE: I remember feeling jealous and angry when other people got pregnant and I couldn't

UE: what if they feel the same about me?

UN: what if they hate me now?

UM: this is really hard

CB: I just want to relax and enjoy it

UA: but I'm scared about so many things

TH: I don't want to jinx anything

IE: I feel confused about who I am now

OE: I have been infertile for so long

UE: my friends and support networks are infertile

UN: I'm in so many infertility groups

UM: should I leave those now?

CB: I can't tell them I'm pregnant

UA: this is really confusing

TH: I just want to be happy about being pregnant

IE: but I feel guilty for being pregnant

OE: and I feel scared that it won't all be okay

UE: what if something goes wrong and I am still infertile?

UN: it feels too soon to hope

UM: I want to be positive, but I'm scared to be

CB: what if something goes wrong?

UA: what if I'm not infertile anymore?

TH: what if I am?

Keep going as long as you need to, being as specific to your circumstances and feelings as you can be.

IE: there's nothing much I can do

OE: except hope

UE: I will be positive

UN: but realistic

UM: I know it's early days

CB: but I know stress doesn't help

UA: so, I'm going to keep myself calm

TH: I'm going to remember to breathe

IE: and I will be quietly hopeful

OE: realistic yet hopeful

UE: I will tell people when I'm ready

UN: and I will trust they will be happy for me

UM: as I'm sure I would be for them

CB: and if I am no longer infertile

UA: I can write a new story

TH: I can inspire others with my story

IE: because if I can get pregnant hopefully, they can too

OE: I have wanted this for so long

UE: and I want to enjoy it

UN: so, for now I will work through my worries

UM: I will be hopeful

CB: I will take care of myself

UA: and I will trust that everything will be okay

TH: I am so happy and grateful to be pregnant.

CHAPTER NINETEEN
ACCEPTING I WILL NEVER BE A MOTHER

"With acceptance comes peace and I am okay."

In some ways this is the most important chapter in this book. You probably started reading this book with hopes of becoming pregnant. But if you've followed all the steps, done everything I've asked of you and yet you're still not pregnant, you may be feeling quite let down and defeated. If this is you, if pregnancy is no longer an option for you, I am so sorry. I had hoped for so much more than this for you.

I have a beautiful friend who is single and has been trying to have a baby now for several years. She has done everything humanly possible to help herself conceive through ART. She has tried Chinese medicine, naturopathy, yoga, essential oils, supplements, diet changes, exercise and medicated ART cycles. All to no avail. While she isn't at acceptance stage yet, as she still has the ability to keep trying more cycles, I tell her story to illustrate that no matter how hard you try, there is always the possibility that you may not be successful in getting the outcome you want.

The only suggestion I can make here is that I believe nothing is random. Everything happens for a reason. I hope one day the reason for your infertility becomes apparent. My journey led me to this book, where will your journey lead you?

One lady told me on the day her final pregnancy attempt failed that she was planning on travelling overseas to consider adoption. In that moment I had a vision of her working in a remote orphanage with kids playing around her and laughing. She too was laughing and looked radiant. I could see her working there for some time, making a big difference in the lives of those children before finding the daughter she would later adopt. She left that day excited for her future and the possibilities it was bringing.

So, you've accepted you will never be pregnant. What do you do now?

First you grieve. Let yourself be sad, angry and anything else you are feeling. You get to feel however you feel and don't let anyone tell you what that should be or low long it should take.

People will make suggestions like fostering and adopting, and these are valid options if they work for you. It is an involved process and, in some ways, can be as emotional and saddening as trying to become pregnant. It might be worth a conversation though. In no way do I believe if you choose to adopt or foster that you are any less of a mother, and I hope they could be options for you to explore in the next part of your story.

This isn't easy, so I send you a world full of love for this process.

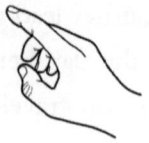

Tapping Script 5: for acceptance

At some point in this journey you may make the decision that you are done trying and accept that motherhood in the traditional sense is not part of your story. You might be okay with this decision if it has been a long time coming and you have had enough. It may be heartbreaking and a decision you never thought you would have to make. The tapping script below is a very general guide. Your feelings around this will be very unique to you. Some of what I write may feel completely aligned with you, and some may not even be in the ball park for you. So, use what you find helpful and change anything that needs to be changed. This script is more directed at people giving up on the idea of having a biological child that they carry.

The karate point (KP): Even though I don't want to give up, I know I have to, and
I love and accept myself deeply and completely.
KP: Even though this is the hardest decision I will ever make I my life,
I love and accept myself deeply and completely.
KP: Even though I know now I won't have a baby,
I love and accept myself deeply and completely.
Inner Eye (IE): this hurts so much

Outer Eye (OE): how do I move on without a baby?

Under Eye (UE): I have spent so much of my life trying

Under Nose (UN): hoping

Under Mouth (UM): how can it be that I'm not a Mum at the end of it?

Collarbone (CB) *use fist*: that I never will be?

Under Arm (UA) *use hand*: is this the right choice?

Top of the head (TH): should I try just once more?

IE: maybe the next time is the one

OE: but I can't live like that

UE: month-after-month not being pregnant

UN: it's too hard

UM: my life has been on hold

CB: I've given up so much already

UA: I need to stop now for my sanity

TH: for my health

IE: this wasn't the outcome I'd hoped for

OE: this wasn't the future I had pictured for myself

UE: I did everything I could

UN: and it wasn't enough

UM: and that hurts

CB: I tried so hard

UA: and I wished it was different

TH: but it's not and it's time to move on

Keep going as long as you need to here ...

IE: I tried as hard as I could

OE: I know in my heart I gave it the best chance

UE: I couldn't have done anymore

UN: it's time to put my energy into something else

UM: there are other areas of my life I have neglected that I would like to focus on now

CB: my relationship needs some TLC

UA: there's new creative projects I'd like to begin

TH: perhaps I could travel

IE: I might go for that promotion I had been outing off

OE: I know I will always have some sadness about not being a Mum

UE: but I'm okay

UN: it will all be okay

UM: I will take each day as it comes

CB: if I feel sad, I will let myself feel sad

UA: if I feel good, I will make the most of it

TH: and the good days will start to outweigh the difficult ones

IE: I am okay

OE: I can do this

UE: I can be okay with this

UN: I love myself and my life

UM: and I'm okay

CB: my life has other plans for me

UA: and it will be great

TH: I am great.

Emotional resources toolkit

Despite doing the exercises throughout this book, perhaps you still have some lingering beliefs or feelings that you are having trouble shifting.

Here are some practical ways of clearing them once and for all!

Affirmations

Using what you have written is a great way to identify your emotions and beliefs that may need changing. Remember, if your new affirmation really doesn't feel believable to you, change the wording to 'I choose…' so that you can believe it, and it gives you an element of control back over how you are feeling. In time you will hopefully find you can remove the 'I choose' altogether.

Put your affirmations on pretty pieces of paper and stick them around the house where you will see them. I have mine on my bathroom mirror, but you might like to put them near your joggers if exercise is a focus for you now, or on the fridge door if you're trying to eat better, maybe on the back of the front door, reminding you to have a great day as you leave the house. Whatever works for you will be fine.

Here is the list of affirmations I have used for the purpose of this book, you might like to change these to suit your specific circumstances:

"I am not defined by my story."

"Today, I take back my power."

"I have the ability to heal myself."

"I connect with the healer within me."

"I commit to showing my body unconditional love and gratitude every day."

"I empower myself with knowledge."

"There are many healthy changes I can make to help me have a baby."

"It is safe to feel my emotions and to listen to what they are telling me."

"I acknowledge and respect my feelings as I work through them."

"I can choose to be the parent I want to be."

"I take responsibility for my energy and my emotions."

"It is safe to examine my emotions."

"My happiness is my responsibility."

"I remind myself to breathe…"

"I am worthy of a healthy and loving relationship."

"Being a mother is my birthright."

"I am grateful for all of the options available to me."

"My past will no longer determine my future."

"I can have a baby while respecting my culture and heritage."

"I am deserving of more than one child."

"I give myself permission to grieve my loss and to move on when I'm ready."

"I am an equal partner in our fertility journey."

"It is okay for me to feel a range of emotions now I'm pregnant."

"With acceptance comes peace and I am okay."

Essential Oils

I have use dōTERRA ClaryCalm to help manage cycles with good effect. A regular cycle is a good step in the right direction on any fertility journey. A few of my favourite oils (or blends) for fertility in women are:

- Copaiba
- Ylang Ylang
- Jasmine
- Melissa
- Rose
- Fennel
- Yarrow
- Geranium
- *Emotional Support: Lavender, Roman Chamomile and Mandarin. (first trimester only)

Essential oils for sperm health may include:

- Frankincense
- Basil
- Cedarwood
- Clary Sage
- Geranium
- Ginger
- Juniper Berry

You can purchase dōTERRA oils through me at www.mydoterra. com/leahlloyd or if you are purchasing elsewhere, please ensure they are of high quality and pure, not synthetic, fragranced oils. I don't have any training in the use of essential oils, so please seek further advice before using them. There are plenty of resources available that can teach you how to use essential oils safely and effectively.

Further Resources

With over fourteen years of experience in nursing, I realised there was often more going on behind-the-scenes with conditions that weren't able to be identified or managed traditionally, leading to my interest in alternative therapies in infertility. To watch my weekly card reading videos, or to read the blog posts, go to:

www.facebook.com/LeahLloydHealer/

www.youtube.com/channelUCbA5BLRdeUoVo9sjoZVibVQ

For further ongoing support, each month I send an email on a different topic and will include a variety of modalities, such as EFT, meditations, card readings, essential oils and other activities **www.leahlloyd.com.**

FORENSIC HEALING

I offer forensic healing sessions in-person or distantly. You can see full details at **www.leahlloyd.com** or visit **www.forensichealing.com** to find a practitioner near you.

EFT

Emotional Freedom Technique or tapping is a great tool for clearing negative beliefs and creating positive ones instead. You can visit **www. thetappingsolution.com** for more information, scripts and videos.

BOOKS

Using Positivity to Make a Better Life by Leah Lloyd.
The Secret Language of Your Body by Inna Segal.
The Low GI Guide to Living Well with PCOS by Dr. Jennie Brand-Miller, M.D.
All available from Amazon in e-book and paperback.

OTHER SERVICES

You may find the help of a naturopath, osteopath, chiropractor, acupuncturist or Chinese medicine beneficial. Ask around in your local area for practitioners that are recommended and others have found helpful in their fertility journey.

Bibliography

Anderson, KN. Ed. 1998, Mosby's Medical, Nursing & Allied Health Dictionary, 5th Edn. Mosby, USA.

The Fertility Society of Australia (2016). http://www.fertilitysociety.com.au/home/about/ [accessed 2/1/16]

Zegers-Hochschild, F., Adamson, GD., de Mouzon, J., Ishihara, O., Mansour, R., Nygren, K., Sullivan, E. and Vanderpoel, S. 2009. *International Committee for Monitoring Assisted Reproductive Technology (ICMART) and the World Health Organisation (WHO) revised glossary of ART terminology, 2009.* http://www.who.int/reproductivehealth/publications/infertility/art_terminology2.pdf?ua=1 [accessed 2/1/16]